Hypnobirth

Parents' Workbook

Transforming Birth Together

The complete antenatal programme

Accredited by the Royal College of Midwives

Teri Gavin-Jones
Sandra Handford

RCM accredited · RCM accredited

All illustrations by Lucy H C Martin, unless otherwise stated.

Cover photo: Spike Grimsey, Rachel Chilver and baby Winnie – hypnobirth family extraordinaire.

ISBN: 978-0-9933732-0-6

First published in 2015 by HypnobirthMidwivesUK

Printed by KGK Creative, 8 & 9 Thundridge Business Park, Cambridge Road, Thundridge, Hertfordshire, SG12 0SS

Preface

HypnobirthMidwivesUK was founded by Teri Gavin-Jones and Sandra Handford. We believe that the combination of hypnotherapy and midwifery results in an evidence-based antenatal course like no other.

The idea behind HypnobirthMidwivesUK is that skilled midwives and other birth professionals are trained to use tried and tested hypnosis and hypnotherapy techniques together with evidence-based midwifery ante-natal training. Together this means that you will receive a Royal College of Midwives (RCM) accredited course, designed by professionals for professionals.

Our aim is to make hypnobirth available to all women and their birthing partners within the NHS. Pregnancy is a life changing event and the more we discover about the way that women birth their babies, the more we realise that childbirth can have a profound impact on the way our babies grow and develop. We understand that birth can be complicated and unpredictable; we feel that women are searching for ways of birthing their babies as naturally, calmly and as easily as possible.

Hypnobirth will enable you to have the best birth possible no matter what happens.

Contents

Welcome to Hypnobirth!

You may know a little or a lot about hypnobirth, but our course aims to inform your decisions around how you would like to birth your baby. We aim to arm you with skills, techniques and strategies that will leave you feeling excited and confident about labour and birth.

Your hypnobirth teacher is also an experienced midwife or birth professional. We believe this combination of hypnobirth and expert knowledge will provide you with all the information you need to make informed choices around birth.

The taught sessions are a complete antenatal course. We are proud to offer the only course that includes hypnosis alongside evidence based birth information. You will learn birth anatomy and physiology from professionals who really know their stuff. The course is logical, medically accurate and research proven.

There are a wide range of antenatal classes available, and we believe that knowledge is power. However if you choose to attend other antenatal classes you may find the philosophy a little different from ours. Hypnobirth uses supportive language, positive affirmations and may encourage you to look at birth differently. A more traditional antenatal class may not offer this, and you may need to keep the hypnobirth philosophy in your mind.

With each session you attend there will be practice to complete. Our expectation is that you work together, in between classes, to achieve the level of relaxation required for a calm birth. This cannot be achieved without practice. Hypnobirth pays great dividends in labour, but only if the work is put in antenatally. Think of it as a gym membership. If you pay your money every month but don't go, you cannot expect to become fit! Signing up alone is not enough. Attending hypnobirth classes alone will not be enough. There is work to be done in between.

The practice is wonderful; your body will thank you for taking time to fit in relaxation. Our couples often say that the time they find to practice the techniques together is very special. Hypnobirth believes that birth partners are crucial to the process. Whoever the birth supporter is, they often want to be fully involved. Our course will provide the birth supporter with essential skills for labour. You will feel fully prepared for your role, and we aim to increase your confidence for the day.

Hypnobirth is for all births. We know that birth does not always go to plan. We have had many successful hypnobirth caesareans, inductions of labour and births that have not been planned for but were the best births possible on the day.

We look forward to working with you towards your best birth.

Section ONE

An Introduction to Hypnobirth

What is Hypnobirth?

Hypnobirth is a way of thinking, an attitude, a philosophy. It is also physical and mental preparation for birth.

Although birth can be described as a natural, instinctive process, western society has medicalised the concept of birth to a point where women feel less confident in their ability to give birth.

Whilst birth intervention rates have risen, there have not been any corresponding improvements in health outcomes. Caesarean rates have increased without any significant change in intrapartum-related perinatal mortality. (CEMACH 2007).

Women and their birth partners are increasingly looking for coping skills and antenatal education that offers a holistic package that is more than the traditional antenatal class.

Hypnobirth offers techniques for any birth experience, including caesarean birth. It encourages couples to remain relaxed and focused whatever path their birth takes.

Hypnobirth combines:

- Deep relaxation techniques
- Breathing techniques for birth
- Understanding how fear and negativity affect the mind and the body
- Visualisation and the use of supportive language
- Knowledge of the birth process
- An understanding of hormones and their role in labour and birth
- The importance of the birth environment
- The importance of the birth partner

What is Hypnosis?

What is hypnosis? Hypnosis is a completely natural state of mind that we experience throughout the day; it's like day-dreaming or meditating. You've probably experienced it when you've driven along a familiar route and you've been thinking about something else and you suddenly notice where you are on your journey. Sometimes people think that they are going to fall asleep during hypnosis and be completely unaware of what is going on, however hypnosis is not sleep.

What does it feel like? It feels like being relaxed. When people first experience hypnosis they often think that nothing is happening. This is because they are thinking that they will be unconscious and won't be able to hear anything. The opposite is true, they will be aware of everything going on around them. Sometimes it feels as if your awareness is expanding, at other times you may become so focussed on a script or a breathing technique that you won't notice anything else around you, this is completely normal. Every time you practice any of the techniques it becomes easier and easier.

Can I be hypnotised? You can only be hypnotised if you want to be. The following people can't be hypnotised effectively:

- Anyone who doesn't want to be hypnotised – this group will often contain very analytical thinkers and those who are reluctant to let go and relax
- The mentally impaired
- People under the influence of alcohol or drugs
- Someone who has little or no understanding of the language being spoken
- Someone who is deaf would be difficult to hypnotise in a group, but on a one-to-one basis hypnosis can be very effective

Can I get stuck in hypnosis? No you can't, hypnosis is a normal brainwave pattern between being fully alert and asleep. You will either become fully alert after hypnosis or you might fall asleep, especially when you are practicing the relaxation techniques just before bedtime.

Will I tell you my deepest secrets or do something daft? Again, the answer is no. A person can only be hypnotised if they want to be, and you will only accept suggestions that you are comfortable with; that fit with your own morals and ethics.

I didn't hear what you were saying, does that matter? Sometimes clients are very tired and fall asleep during relaxation. Sometimes they are simply in a deep trance and although they haven't consciously heard what's been said they still follow the instructions to come back into the room and open their eyes. This means that they will have taken in all the other suggestions made to them.

I've never heard the end of the CD, is that OK? The CD has been written for relaxation and if couples are listening to it when they're in bed and it is helping them to have a good night's sleep, then that is all to the good. Sometimes mums are worried that they are asleep before they hear the affirmations; this track can be listened to whilst pottering about the house. You might be able to make time during the day to listen to the whole CD. The CD is powerful. Do not listen to it whilst driving.

Can I talk in hypnosis? You can communicate when you are in a hypnotic state. Very often we will use finger movements or a nod of the head. This keeps you from re-engaging the neocortex and helps you to stay in 'the zone'. Some types of hypnotherapy use a very light trance which allows the therapist and client to talk. This type of work is often used to examine past events and explore future possibilities. We don't usually use this in hypnobirth because we want the mother to be as deeply relaxed as possible where talking would be too much of an effort unless absolutely necessary.

Will I be unreachable? Even if a person is so deeply relaxed that they don't hear very much of what's being said, they will usually respond to an instruction. For example, at the end of the scripts you will be invited to bring your attention back into the room and to notice your fingers and toes and perhaps to have a little stretch. Most people will do exactly that when the suggestion is made. Of course, sometimes you might fall asleep.

Something I have noticed over many years of working with clients is that if there is a part of a script or CD that they don't like they won't hear it no matter how many times they listen to it – it's almost as if the brain blocks that particular instruction! As we've already mentioned, you will only accept suggestions that you are comfortable with.

Exercise: Make a note of any questions you'd like to ask about hypnosis...

The Power of the Mind

In his book *The Wizard Within*, Dr Al Krasner, who was a world-renowned hypnotherapist and teacher, used the analogy of the robot. He said that if we were a robot the brain/mind would be the computer and that every thought that we have has a physical effect on the body. Krasner named his book after the wizard in the Wizard of Oz. He believed that our mind is the 'wizard' and that every thought we have causes a physical response in the body.

The brain/computer also reacts to external influences before the brain has consciously noticed the cause. For example, you notice that you are feeling cold and decide to close the window, but what happened before you realised that you were feeling chilly. At first your brain/computer will have registered the temperature gradually beginning to drop and it makes adjustments to your circulation, moving the blood supply away from the skin and the extremities to conserve heat in the core so that your organs continue to function. This, in turn, causes a physical reaction on the surface of the skin and, when the reaction is large enough, the conscious part of the mind will notice that you are feeling cold and you will get up and close the window.

Although we have always known that the body reacts to our thoughts this is now supported by neuroscience. Award-winning, pioneering neuroscientist Richard J Davidson states in his book *The Emotional Life of your Brain* that "*Feelings and thoughts, which originate in the brain, literally get out of that grey matter and into the rest of the body*." He explains that "*modern neuroscience has shown that emotions do infuse not only the mind but also the body. Feeling anxious raises your blood pressure and makes your pulse race, and feeling content can strengthen your immune system...*"

Here are some examples of a thought causing a physical reaction:

- Fingernails screeching across a blackboard – does that set your teeth on edge?

- Fear – If you are afraid of spiders or snakes and you imagine one moving towards your foot. How does your body respond?
- Hunger – does your mouth water or your tummy rumble just by thinking about food?
- Sex – for men, a very obvious physical response to a sexy thought!
- Anxiety – a job interview, giving a presentation in front of colleagues; if it's important and you need to get it right, maybe your heart rate increases at the thought. Do your palms get a little sweaty?

If we think of the mind as an iceberg, the conscious mind would be the tip of the iceberg. The conscious part of the mind is where we do all of our analytical thinking; where we make our day to day decisions; where we make judgements and where willpower resides.

The unconscious part of the mind, however, stores all our memories, habits and is responsible for the running of our bodies, e.g. your digestion, circulation, hormones, etc. The conscious part of the mind can do between 3 and 5 things at once, whilst the unconscious part of the mind processes vast amounts of information all of the time.

So in a contest between the conscious and unconscious parts of the mind, no matter how much will power we use the unconscious part of the mind will eventually win. This is why hypnosis is so successful for changing habits and for assisting us to make the positive changes in our lives that we desire. The techniques that you will learn during this course are often used by athletes to improve sports performance; by students working to pass important exams; and for many other life skills.

In order for a new skill to become a habit you must practice it over and over again. Just as you did when you were learning to ride a bike, or drive a car. To begin with you had to think about what you were doing and concentrate, focussing your attention on the details. Then you practiced and practiced until it became a habit. You no longer needed to think about how to ride a bike or drive a car. It is the same with the techniques that you will learn in your hypnobirth classes. In between classes, as you practice together, you will both learn new positive habits to enable you to feel confident and empowered during the birth of your baby.

Another great advantage of these techniques is that they translate well from hypnobirth for use in all sorts of areas of your life.

One of the most important things to remember about the mind is that the thoughts that we have can become our reality, especially thoughts that are charged with energy and power. The more emotion there is attached to a thought, the more powerful it can become. If we have two opposite thoughts or feelings about an event, the thought with the strongest emotion attached to it will inevitably win.

Recently I was staying in a hotel and was chatting with one of the members of staff, a very friendly girl called Aggie. I asked Aggie whether she was working the following day and she pulled a bit of a face and said that she was on the early shift which meant that she would have to get up at 6:30am. Now Aggie was very energetic and efficient, but didn't really like early mornings, and never slept very well the night before. When I asked her why, she told me that she worried that she wouldn't wake up on time. So the evening before the thoughts going through her head were "I won't wake up, I'm going to be late. What if I don't hear the alarm? I'll get into trouble". These thoughts would whir around her head until eventually she would fall asleep only to wake a few hours later to repeat these same thoughts. This would typically happen two or three more times before she had to get up, feeling tired and lethargic. I suggested that she might like to try something different. Instead of her usual thoughts, she should simply say "I will wake at 6:30, I will wake at 6:30, I will wake at 6:30", and if she awoke in the night to repeat it again as she quickly fell asleep.

The next morning I went down to breakfast and was greeted by a grinning Aggie who told me that she had done as I suggested and had had the best night's sleep she'd had in ages, and had woken up at 6:30am on the dot feeling fantastic! She had told all the other members of staff on duty who wanted to know if I had any other tips for tiredness and insomnia! Incidentally I also woke at 6:30am because I had neglected to change the thought in my own mind after explaining the process to Aggie – I think that comes under the heading of "be careful what you wish for..."

Something else you may have noticed in the suggestion that I gave Aggie is that it was positively expressed. By that I mean that instead of saying "I won't oversleep, I won't oversleep, I won't oversleep" I suggested that she said "I will wake at 6:30" and so on. The reason for this is that the mind doesn't do negatives. If I say to you "don't think of a pink elephant" what image immediately comes into your mind?

I used to have a colleague who would go to the local shop each day to get his lunch and often someone would say "don't forget the milk" and invariably he would come back without milk. I explained about the brain and negatives and once the instruction was changed to "remember the milk", invariably he would. Try this at home with family or friends and see what happens!

This is important when you are using affirmations or talking about your pregnancy, labour and birth. Keep your new thoughts, affirmations and stories positive. This can feel awkward to begin with as you become aware of how much negative language you use and stories you tell yourself. Simply notice and begin to change to a more positive frame of mind.

Now that you are ready to begin to choose new positive thoughts to replace and release the old negative ones, the next exercise will help you to develop your new habits and beliefs.

Part 1: Think about some of the thoughts that go through your mind about pregnancy and birth that you would like to change, and write them down on the next page.

Old NEGATIVE thoughts and ideas:

Part 2: Write three new affirmations now. Choose positive language, which will lead to different actions and behaviours, and with practice these become your new habits and beliefs. Begin the change today!

Three new POSITIVE affirmations:

REMEMBER:

To change how you are feeling about something, begin by changing your thoughts

Use positive language

Keep your new affirmation in the present tense otherwise it will remain in the future

Repeat it over and over again until it becomes your new belief

If you notice yourself falling back into old habits, simply notice and change to the new affirmation or thought

The Use of Language in Hypnobirth

"Words are, of course, the most powerful drug used by mankind." Rudyard Kipling

Why do we change our words for hypnobirth?

It is important to understand the power of language.

Research tells us that the way we respond to words, and language, can produce a physical, and emotional, response in our bodies.

Positive language makes us strong and powerful, you only have to listen to someone talking about a topic that they are passionate about. They will use positive words and be filled with positive energy and enthusiasm; this is infectious and has a powerful impact on the recipient.

Negative language has the opposite effect. Consider how you feel when you listen to someone who talks negatively about themselves, or their work or their personal life. It can leave you feeling down and drained of energy. Have you ever experienced 'the moaner' at work? The person who is dissatisfied, unhappy, and demotivated. The moaner will complain to anyone who listens. Sadly there is a tendency for others to join in. Before you know it there is a whole group of moaners. Negativity, as well as positivity spreads.

This kind of negative language eventually turns into a self fulfilling prophecy. Negative words affect the physiology, and emotions, setting limits on what we believe we can achieve.

Words can have an impact on our feelings, our emotions, and enable or disable us. Consider the following sentence spoken to a woman in labour by a midwife:

"When I examined you, you were only 4cms dilated"

It is the word **ONLY** that will affect the woman.

Small words can change the entire feel of a conversation:

"I'm **just** a stay at home mum"

"I'm **still** in the same job"

Reframing is a technique we use in hypnobirth. It is simply taking a negative thought and standing it on its head so that it becomes a positive one. It is exactly the same technique as pointing out that a half empty glass is also half full. This is a conversational Neuro Linguistic Programming (NLP) technique and is not hypnosis, but can be used under hypnosis to make a positive reframe. It is also a powerful way to train yourself or another to think positively. Birth partners are important reframers, and will be able to assist the woman to reframe any negative thoughts around birth.

The language used by birth professionals can be both confusing and a little overwhelming.

Words are an important form of communication. If your care provider is using medical jargon or abbreviations then your understanding of the situation can be limited. The hypnobirth language aims to use clearly identifiable terms. If there is no substitute we will clearly explain the medical terminology in class.

Section ONE Summary

- Hypnosis is a normal state of mind
- You can only be hypnotised if you want to be
- You will only follow suggestions that you are comfortable with
- Hypnosis enhances feelings of calm, confidence and relaxation
- You can't get stuck in hypnosis
- The unconscious mind is incredibly powerful
- Professional athletes use visualisation and breathing techniques to improve performance
- Habits are formed by repeating an action (or a technique) over and over again
- Beliefs are formed by repeating a thought over and over again
- Your thoughts create a physical response in your body
- Change your thoughts, your language, and your actions to create new beliefs and habits
- You mind does not do negatives, so keep your language and thoughts positive
- Every time you listen to the CD or a script, it becomes easier and easier. So practice, practice, practice!

Section TWO

The Biology of Birth

Breathing for Birth

Notice how small children breathe. Watch as their stomach moves with the breath. This is called abdominal breathing.

As we breathe in, we should see the stomach rise slightly as the dome of the diaphragm contracts and compresses the abdominal space. As we breathe out, both the chest and the stomach fall. If you look at young children, this is what you usually see.

Now check your breathing. As adults we often breathe in and the chest rises as the intercostal muscles contract. When this happens the stomach is drawn in. Our modern lifestyle contributes to this type of shallow breathing. It may even start from as early as when children first go to school and have to sit on a chair leaning over a desk or table. Poor posture makes abdominal breathing difficult; slouching on a sofa doesn't help either!

For women especially we are very used to holding onto our abdominal muscles. Body image may have a negative impact on our ability to breathe deeply. A flat stomach is seen as desirable and therefore the breath has moved into shallow chest breathing. This type of breathing reduces the volume of oxygen available as it only partly expands the lungs.

The hypnobirth breath is called ***surge breathing***, and is essentially abdominal breathing.

This exercise will help you to engage the diaphragm and focus on your breathing.

- Lie on the floor face up with knees slightly bent. Place a small pillow under the head if that is more comfortable for you
- Place your hands lightly on your stomach your finger tips just touching

- Concentrate on breathing using the diaphragm, not using the chest, and feeling the stomach rise as the lungs fill from the bottom
- As you breathe in your fingertips should no longer touch
- Let the stomach fall naturally when breathing out by relaxing the diaphragm

Why do we need to learn breathing techniques for labour? It is simple, your labour and birth is a physical and emotional journey. It will probably be the hardest work of your life. It is incredibly rewarding, but will require all your focus. Just as for any physical challenge you will need to prepare. All sportsmen and women use breathing techniques. They realise the importance of gaining the most from their bodies using the breath available. Birth is a physical challenge, and the correct breathing will maximise oxygen to both you and your baby. It releases tension in the uterus and can steady your pulse and stabilize blood pressure.

When we experience a new sensation, such as labour, it can cause us to respond with tension. When your body is tense the muscles constrict and your breathing is shallow. Your oxygen levels are reduced. This makes performing any physical task, including labour, more difficult.

Slow breathing triggers the relaxation response. Muscles are relaxed and oxygenated, blood pressure reduces, your heart rate slows and physical tasks are easier to perform.

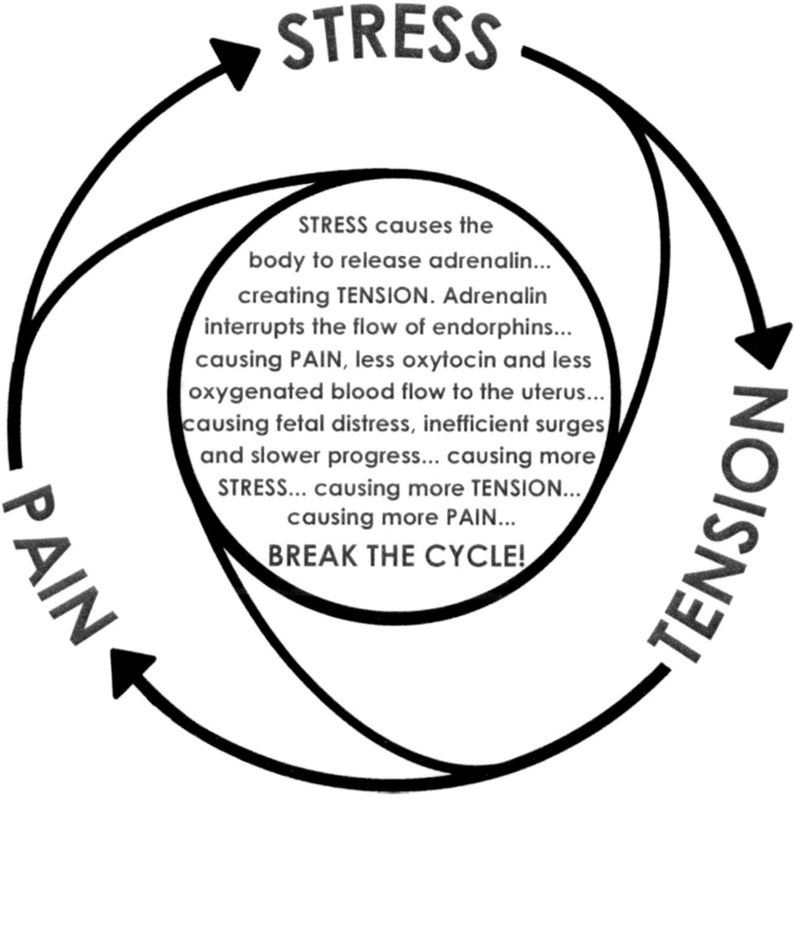
STRESS
TENSION
PAIN
STRESS causes the
body to release adrenalin...
creating TENSION. Adrenalin
interrupts the flow of endorphins...
causing PAIN, less oxytocin and less
oxygenated blood flow to the uterus...
causing fetal distress, inefficient surges
and slower progress... causing more
STRESS... causing more TENSION...
causing more PAIN...
BREAK THE CYCLE!

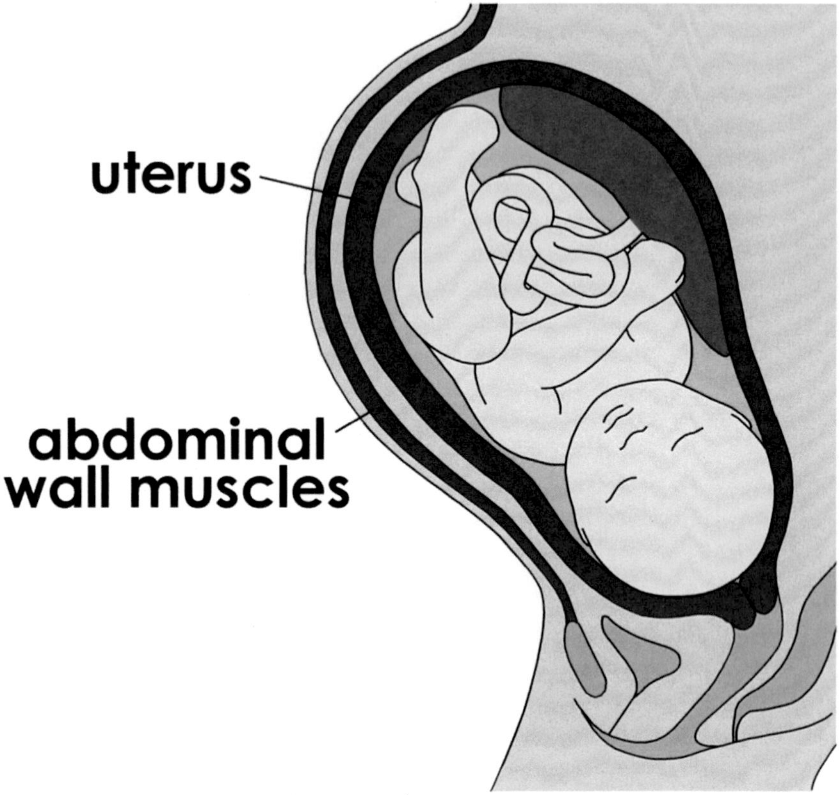

The uterus in pregnancy is a large muscle. When a woman experiences a surge the uterus becomes tight. If this tightness – the contracting – feels painful, the woman often tenses. She may hold her breath. By doing so she is also tensing the abdominal wall which is covering the uterus. We now have two tight tense muscle layers. Does it increase any pain? Yes. Surge breathing delivers extra oxygen to the uterus and the baby, relaxes the abdominal wall and releases tension. The surge becomes manageable.

Surge Breathing Practice

Find somewhere comfortable and quiet to sit

Close your eyes and be mindful of your breath. Begin inhaling through the nose, and as you do mentally slowly count to 3

As you exhale through the mouth count to 6

Continue to breathe in, inflating the abdomen to a slow count of 3

Continue to breathe out deflating the abdomen to a count of 6

You may notice a natural pause at the end of the out breath

Just rest in the space. Wait for the in breath to come of its own accord

Inhale – 3

Exhale – 6

As you train your body to slow breathe you may find your count changes. It may lengthen to 4 and 8, or even 5 and 10

Practice is the key!

Alex's story

I was perhaps in a slightly unusual position in that my husband did not wish to attend the birth. He is not comfortable in hospitals and we both agreed that it would be better to have someone there who could support me.

Instead, my cousin acted as my birth partner. She was very experienced after three children of her own but was arguably sceptical about hypnobirthing, having never done it herself. Unfortunately, we couldn't rehearse the exercises together between sessions so I listened to the CDs and practiced the breathing every day on my own, mainly when I went to bed.

In the meantime, she planned what she would bring/do to support me based on what I liked best during the sessions, for example, certain types of touch, visualisation or anchoring. I found there were definitely some which I responded better to than others and which I would listen to repeatedly, usually falling asleep before I got to the end!

Despite some initial worries that I wouldn't be able to find the time to practice every day, I found that it slotted in quite easily to my routine.

In fact, I used the techniques on numerous occasions when there was stress at work, on the train home after a hectic day, going to bed and during a procedure to remove an abscess. It was during the latter that I noticed the breathing really helped me manage what was some of the worst pain I have experienced. By the time I was 40 weeks, I was having regular Braxton Hicks and started to use the breathing to get through them.

Hormones and Birth

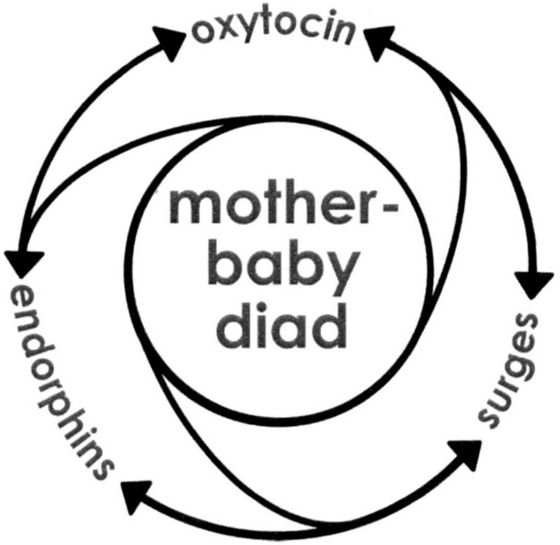

Birth is dominated by a cocktail of hormones. When labour begins the body releases oxytocin. This is received by oxytocin receptors in the uterus, which in turn produces the surge.

The baby also produces oxytocin.

Oxytocin is the power behind a labour. It produces and maintains the surge. This balance needs to be nurtured for labour to continue.

Oxytocin is stored in the anterior pituitary and released in pulses every 3-5 minutes in early labour. This is a rhythm that the smooth muscles of the uterus respond to, and establishes regular surges. The spaces between the surges are just as important as the surges themselves. This is the time when your body adds another hormone – beta-endorphins. Endorphins are similar in effect to opiates, but naturally produced. They activate the mesocorticolimbic dopamine reward system, producing feelings of pleasure. Endorphins increase tolerance to pain, and make whole experience manageable.

Oxytocin is an essential hormone in all aspects of our lives. When forming relationships with other people oxytocin plays a role. It enhances what is called 'social memory'. It can enable us to prefer certain individuals over another. When we meet someone with whom we feel a 'spark', it is oxytocin we are feeling. In all female mammals it allows a mother to learn to recognize and prefer her own offspring. This is why babies produce their own oxytocin, to ensure the mother-baby bonding process.

Oxytocin is an intimate hormone. It responds best to environmental and emotional influences. Couples produce large amounts of oxytocin when they make love. It is this that gives us a wonderful sense of fulfilment. To set the scene for romance and intimacy, and to allow the oxytocin to peak, there may be some environmental influences that can encourage or discourage intimacy.

Privacy – being able to relax is essential. Disruptions and disturbances interrupt the oxytocin flow. You are more likely to relax in an environment that is quiet, warm and softly lit. Oxytocin responds to our senses, so smells, music, good food and touch will all increase it.

Can you begin to see how important the role of oxytocin is in labour, and how it can be increased or decreased?

The birth environment can impact a great deal on your oxytocin levels. Begin to think about early labour. What can you do at home to increase oxytocin?

Rachel's story

After examination I discovered I was 9cm dilated. As I continued to breathe through the surges with some sacral massage, the birthing pool was filled, the lights dimmed and the star projector created an amazing calming effect that filled the room. I felt safe and ready. Chris placed our LED candles around the space and the relaxation music used in class was playing on my iPod.

The Birth Environment

"The external environment dictates the internal environment" - Uvnas-Moberg (2003)

Where you give birth, the environment and who supports your birth are all essential elements for a good labour to happen. For women with complex pregnancies, there may little choice and the obstetric environment will be the obvious one. For straightforward pregnancies there are more options. Since the 1960s and '70s, birth in hospital has risen until today it is where the majority of women give birth. To enable the easiest birth you must choose the location where you feel the most comfortable and relaxed. That could be at home, in a midwifery led unit or an obstetric unit. As your pregnancy progresses your initial ideas may change. This is fine, and your place of birth can be changed at any time.

Birth is instinctive, intimate and private. Yet the expectation is that women do it in a public building, supported by a midwife who is often new to you. Although on a conscious level this is a logical choice, your biological mammalian brain will find this challenging. It will help if you have a comfortable space where you can relax, and often this is not the bed. This can feel too clinical, and will result in restricting movement. Hospital rooms can lack the softness of home. The birth partner can create a nest using a floor mat, beanbag, birth ball and your own pillow.

Hospitals are busy places. Sometimes equipment that is in your room may be needed elsewhere. It may result in a different midwife requesting something, or asking your midwife a question. Hypnobirth techniques are valuable in training you to focus and not let other sounds/interruptions disturb you. At all times the person making the request should knock and wait for a response. The midwife or birth partner can then go to the door. Having people enter the room without being invited is unacceptable.

Maternity units are realising the importance of maintaining the environment and have come a long way in adjusting the birth environment. They know the benefits of oxytocin release, and the impact the environment has on it.

What can help?

- Darkness – dim the lights, dimmer switch, lamp
- LED candles
- Change the smell – aromatherapy oils?
- Music
- Hypnobirth CD
- Warm temperature
- Bed to the side of the room
- Alternative furniture – bean bag, birth ball, mats, rocking chair, birth stool
- Privacy and quiet
- Offer hydrotherapy – pool/bath/shower
- Encourage nest building
- Keep the pelvis upright and mobile
- Consider Rebozo
- Massage
- Breathing techniques
- Lovely food
- Your own pillow/throw/duvet

Birth partner, your role is to keep the oxytocin high if you move from home to hospital.

Exercise: Begin a list of what you will need to achieve total relaxation in your birth room

Adrenalin, Fear and Birth

Adrenalin is a hormone produced when we perceive stress, fear or threat. It creates a mammalian 'fight or flight' response. This can mean survival for many mammals, but when it occurs within a birth environment it can mean a stall in labour.

The production of adrenalin can be initiated by something very obvious, or completely subtle.

How do you feel about hospitals? What do you associate with a hospital? Is it sickness, injury, death? For many women pregnancy and birth are normal physiological events. If you have added complexities then you will need the support of the hospital and the medics. However most women are fit and well, therefore being in a hospital can feel a little odd.

Birth is instinctive, intimate and private. Yet the expectation is that we do it in a public building. These are the reasons many maternity units have come a long way in adjusting the birth environment. They know the benefits of oxytocin release, and the impact the environment has on it.

When a woman is producing oxytocin, she is in the relaxed response. When she is producing adrenalin she is initiating a stress response.

In the boxes we can see the physiological effect of the different hormones on the body.

Hypnobirth and a great birth partner can keep the woman in the relaxed response.

The Stress Response

- Increased adrenalin
- Constricted pupils
- Increased heart rate
- Raised blood pressure
- Quick, shallow breathing
- Tense, tight muscles

The Relaxed Response

- Increased oxytocin
- Dilated pupils
- Slow and steady heart rate
- Lower blood pressure
- Slow, deep breathing
- Loose, relaxed muscles

Sensation in Labour

Some hypnobirth courses promise a pain free birth. There have been women who have contacted us after labour and talked about a pain free experience. Most women experience sensation in labour, some a lot, some a little. We do not know what kind of sensations you will experience in labour. However we do know that our hypnobirth course will make your experience more comfortable.

There are women who will tell you that labour is the most painful thing they have ever experienced. There are also women who give birth and feel very little sensation. Others give birth and describe it as euphoric. We have heard and seen both ends of the spectrum. What we can say with certainty is that all women tell us that hypnobirth improved their experience.

So why is it that some women feel intense sensations, whilst others can feel none?

Jody's story

All those months of worry and it was a pain free and a wonderful birth. I wish I had enjoyed my pregnancy more and stopped stressing over the birth.

Hypnobirth was incredible and a massive contributing factor in to how I was home within 10 hours of arriving in to the hospital. I cannot thank you enough or explain how much this has been life changing. Thank you.

Cultural influences

Anthropologist Margaret Mead noted that, depending on the culture, birth is seen as being either a painful and dangerous event or an interesting, enriching experience. Some cultures tolerate the expression of pain; in others it is not acceptable at all.

Our western culture is often focused on fixing pain. If we have a headache we may reach for the pain killers. It might have been useful to track back the cause of the headache; dehydration, stress, neck tension, eye strain. Instead of solving the underlying cause, we often look for a quick fix. Medical advances have evolved to a point where it seems pointless to suffer. This attitude may be absolutely right for illness, but can we apply it to birth sensations? Does it need fixing?

Anthropological studies into childbirth suggest that there are societies that live in harmony with nature and its rhythms and have a greater understanding of birth – the instinctive model.

Industrialised societies such as ours, live an intense lifestyle geared to productivity. There is no room for rhythm. We are time and goal orientated, and this often includes birth.

Physiological events are expected to take place in a linear fashion. We can see this from the medical model of birth. Dilatation is supposed to happen in a linear fashion, from 0–10 cm, and within a certain timeframe.

In reality the female body establishes a rhythm that may not perform to text book definitions. Instead of accepting that all women and babies are individual; we blame the woman's body if she does not conform to the medical parameters, and call it 'failure to progress'. Thus labelling her a failure and birth as impossible.

There are cultures that celebrate not only birth but the female journey. As a woman we experience many physical changes which some cultures see as 'rites of passage'.

These big events for a woman can be:

- First menstrual bleed
- Puberty
- Childbirth
- Breastfeeding
- Menopause

How as a society do we view these issues? Menstruation is a topic that is still not often discussed. There are entire supermarket isles devoted to what is known as 'sanitary wear'. Is this because we view it as unsanitary? There are products to enable women to wipe, douche and cleanse ourselves. The words 'fragrance' and 'odour free' are often used; implying that this time of the month is dirty, somehow unclean. One feminist blogger writes *"Don't get me started on the advert for Tampax, wherein your period is depicted as 'Mother Nature', a prudish hag in a twinset who keeps trying to ruin your fun at a music festival, thus implying that women are in constant battle with the completely natural processes of their bodies"*. (Bourne 2014)

How does society view childbirth within our culture? Many years ago birth was an event that took place in the community. It was supported by other women, the midwife, but also mothers, sisters, aunts and friends. Women supported other women through birth, and the event was a normal part of life. Today we have moved birth into the hospital, and for many women this is the appropriate place. However it has become shrouded in mystery. The only time women can now see births is on TV, and it has been turned into entertainment. TV births are often dramatic and heavily edited. This voyeuristic view of childbirth only increases women's fear. Many of the TV births are bed bound and often 'fixed' with drugs. This portrayal feeds women's fear surrounding birth.

Other female bodily functions to be 'improved' upon are breastfeeding and the menopause. Both can be fixed, one with formula and the other with HRT.

Now we are not suggesting for a moment that we all embrace menstruation, birth our babies in tents and turn into militant breastfeeding earth mothers (unless that suits you!). However we do suggest paying close attention to the messages we receive from advertising and the media. It is important that we, as women, unpick how society and the media portray our bodily functions.

Interestingly, there are also cultures where male rites of passage take place. These rituals can involve men voluntarily subjecting themselves to physical or psychological tests and challenges, as it is seen to make them stronger and more powerful when they survive. In this context such feats of endurance can be seen as positive.

Expectation of birth

A study in 1993 looked at 700 women and their expectation of birth (Green, 1993). It concluded that women tended to experience what they expected to, whether that was a lot of sensation or a little. Even women who have not experienced birth before had already decided it was going to be painful. This may be as a result of media portrayal, friends and relatives' birth stories, or the cultural expectation as previously discussed.

What we do know is that your mind is a powerful influence on your body's performance. Just consider any challenging physical task. A marathon runner will tell you that at some point, usually 20 miles, they hit 'the wall'. As well as physical, they will often talk about the mental energy that is needed to sustain such a challenge. Sports psychologists use visualisations and positive affirmations when training. If an athlete continually believes they cannot win the race, chances are they will lose. This same level of expectation of success must be used in pregnancy as expectancy is a powerful tool.

Physical sensation

Some women experience intense physical sensations during childbirth. Others do not. We must ask ourselves, if women all have a womb and a baby, how can experiences be so different?

Sensation emanates from two sources – the physical body and the brain. Both work together to produce an individual experience for that person. Let's look at the brain first.

The Affective-Motivational Dimension

This is based in the thalamus of the brain, it is the part of the brain that relays sensory information from the body into the brain. It allows the woman to interpret where she feels a sensation, what it feels like, and its intensity.

What can we do to influence it?

- Surge Breathing
- Massage
- Hydrotherapy –birth pool, shower
- Hot and cold – hot water bottle/ice packs

The Emotional Dimension

This is found in the limbic system; it receives the information about sensations and allocates them an emotional value. It is receptive to the neocortex (the 'thinking' part of your brain).

What can we do to influence it?

It can be altered with external conditions such as the environment.

- Soft lighting
- Music
- Smells
- Feeling safe and unobserved,

The Cognitive-Evaluating Dimension

This depends on information, and is influenced by cultural experiences and our perspective of sensations. It can activate or inhibit both other dimensions of sensation.

What can we do to influence it?

- Understand how culture, media and society influence our preconceptions about birth.
- Education
- Hypnosis
- Abdominal breathing

(Schmid, 2011)

What are the Physical Factors that can Increase a Woman's Sensations?

- Breath holding/ anxiety breathing
- Muscle tension
- Fatigue
- Dehydration, lack of food
- Poor positions – lying on her back
- Position of the baby

Claire's story

Albert (Bertie) was born on Monday 25th May weighing 7lb 10oz. We had a natural birth in a birthing pool using hypnobirth, gas and air and paracetemol (I think the paracetemol was just placebo on my part.) My labour started on Sunday lunchtime but I didn't realise that's what it was until about midnight, Chris popped me in the bath with some aromatherapy oil burning and my hypno CD.

There were only a couple of times when I doubted myself but Chris quickly brought me round and your voice kept on popping into my head too. It was really special for both me and Chris but one of the most special things is that Bertie was born in his own waters with the sack still intact. Once he'd arrived our midwife opened his sack and he floated up into my arms, a moment we will never forget. Everything went quiet, and I felt like there was only me, Chris and Bertie in the world.

We never realised before doing the hypnobirthing that labour could be such a positive experience for both me and Chris and we cannot thank you enough for that, we're pretty evangelical about it.

Birth sensation can be seen as an initiation, a means of personal change or transformation. We could decide to use it, work with it, know that the sensations in labour are normal. There are those of course who prefer not to feel the sensation of labour. Can birth be 'fixed'? Can we remove all sensation and enjoy a sensation free birth? There are drugs available, and what you need to know is that just because you are doing a hypnobirth course it does not have to be a drug free birth.

We want you to feel informed, empowered and in control. The reality is that the choice of drugs available to a labouring woman and her child are limited. Certainly you have tried to avoid many things during pregnancy – any drug stronger than paracetamol, alcohol, caffeine, unpasteurised food. In labour it is difficult to administer strong pain killers that work well yet do not affect the baby.

Epidural anaesthesia is often seen as the most effective form of pain management. However there are some down sides. Labour sensation is unique because of its rhythmic nature. Due to the contrast between peaks of sensation and absolute sensation-free spaces, endorphins are produced.

Endorphins reduce the experience of sensation and induce a feeling of fulfilment, well-being and euphoria. They also promote bonding with your baby. When we introduce intervention such as an epidural, the physiology of birth has to change. Epidural inhibits endorphin production. It also inhibits oxytocin levels in labour which can slow or stop labour. There is an oxytocin peak that usually occurs at the time of birth which is triggered by stretching the receptors of the woman's lower vagina. These are numbed by the epidural which is why second stage labour can be much longer and may need assistance with forceps or ventous.

When the sensation of labour is removed by epidural, the body can think the surges are no longer needed. Physiologically the body thinks it is no longer in labour and the surges begin to slow down. This combined with having to remain lying down can slow or stop birth.

We can see from the spiral below that the body relies on the labour sensation to produce the appropriate hormones.

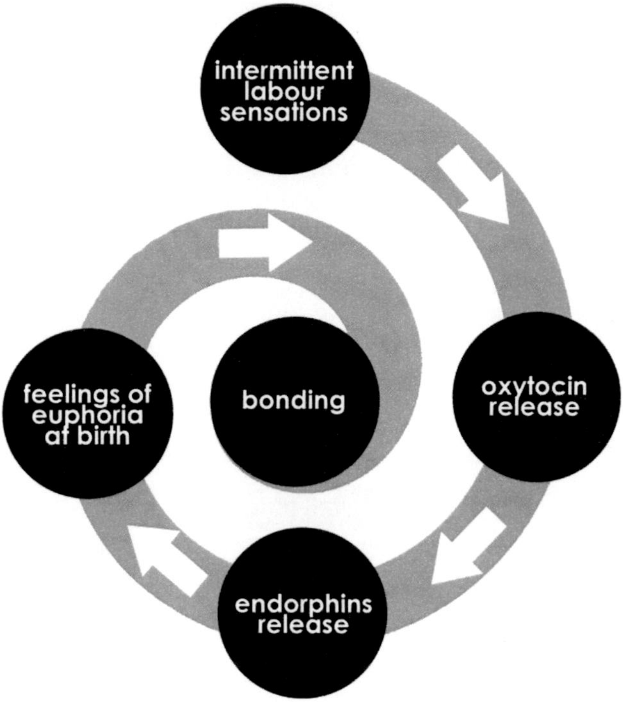

Not all epidurals are effective, and many women are unaware that there is any failure rate. If the epidural is seen by the woman as something to enable her to cope, something she is pinning her hopes on, and then it is ineffective, where else is there to go?

We need a full range of coping skills for birth. The failure rate for epidural is small, and it is difficult to assess 'failure'. Sara Wickham explains *"pain and pain relief are subjective and people have different expectations, the definition of 'success' will vary between people, including researchers. To put it into research terms, there is no universal outcome measure for this. Does an epidural have to remove every last smidgen of sensation to be successful, or is it still a success if it removes 90 per cent of pain but the woman is OK with that?"* (www.sarawickham.com 2014)

The best data suggests there is a failure rate of 23% (Thangamuthu et al 2013). This still involves some uncertainties but it is clearly difficult to assess definitive figures.

Whenever we rely on sources that are external we must prepare ourselves for variation. An epidural can be absolutely appropriate for some women. However the epidural 'solution' often means a woman must behave passively during a potentially creative event. A medicalised labour and birth inhibits the production of hormones. It does not allow the woman to experience the profound fulfilment of the birthing experience. The wish to repeat the experience is dramatically reduced. The bonding is affected. The labour experience becomes a traumatic event that is retold – thus compounding the horror stories of birth.

It is important that you are well informed when making decisions around childbirth and that all information is available to you. We as hypnobirth practitioners support your choices in labour. Our aim is not to judge, but to ensure you are fully informed. Birth does not always go to plan and intervention has its place. Whatever happens will be your 'best birth'.

Becky's story

It wasn't until near the very end that I felt the need for a little gas and air (I think that may have been because it was all so quick) but I certainly wouldn't have needed any other pain relief. The breathing techniques, positive thinking and visualisations were what got me through it. It may sound strange but in my mind I knew that I wouldn't need any sort of intervention because I was so confident about what I had to do, I had planned it in my mind and all I had to do was put it into practice.

Claire and Andy's story

The hypnobirth classes made an incredible difference to my labour and also my pregnancy. I was so frightened of the labour process, but once I started the hypnobirth course I fully embraced it and actually looked forward to labour. It totally changed mine and my husband's attitude and changed my focus to looking forward to having my baby, rather than being scared of the labour.

The hypnobirth course took the fear out of labour and I felt it gave me a lot of control over my own labour and pregnancy. My husband (who has a terrible fear of hospitals) also found the course incredibly helpful and empowering. Initially he feared he would not be able to be there with me during labour, but having done the course, he was the most supportive and encouraging and calm birth partner I could have hoped for.

If hypnobirth can offer the benefit of reducing labour sensation without the associated complications of pharmacological analgesia, then logic tells us it is beneficial. Much research into hypnobirth has focused on the use of analgesia for labour. However hypnobirth offers a multifaceted range of benefits, and couples report time and again their experience of hypnobirth:

- Shorter labours
- Less use of drugs
- Reduced hospital stay
- Increased relationship closeness antenatally during the practice

- More likely to experience normal birth
- Full birth partner involvement
- Feelings of confidence
- Reduced risk of postnatal depression
- Calmer babies
- Better family bonding

Mammalian Birth

Often when talking about birth we might start to compare human birth to other species. We may wonder why other animals do not seem to suffer in the same way female humans do in childbirth.

As your pregnancy progresses, and you begin to anticipate the day your baby will be born, you may begin to doubt your ability to birth easily, naturally or without medical intervention. Do you suppose there are other mammals out there with the same doubts? Do you see your heavily pregnant cat fretting that she may not be able to birth her babies? Do elephants question their ability to birth?

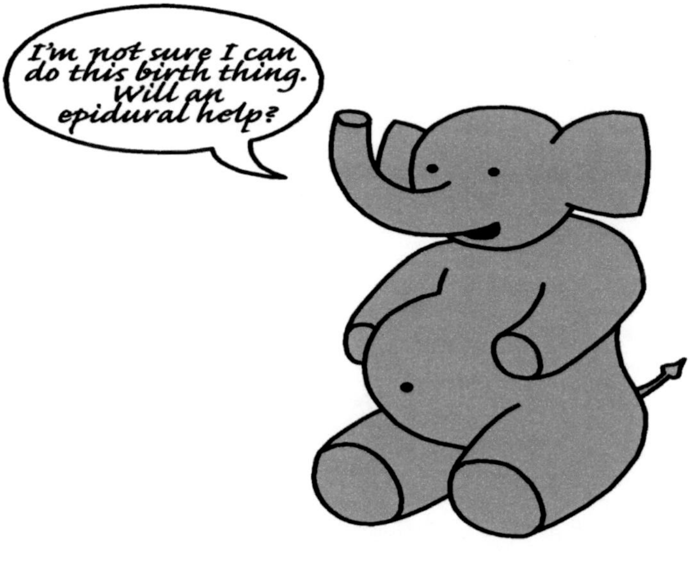

We are the only mammals who doubt our own ability to birth our babies. Does this get in the way of birth? Probably. The reason we are able to question, doubt and worry about birth is the function of our enlarged neocortex. The neocortex is the 'thinking' part of our brain. It is this evolutionary difference that separates us from other mammals.

The neocortex is where we analyse, rationalise and question. The primal brain is where bodily functions such as birth take place. For birth to happen swiftly and spontaneously the woman must use her primal brain. We will often hear woman describing being 'zoned out' or 'on another planet' in labour. Women find themselves adopting instinctive positions, using primal noises, sweating, swaying, grunting and immersing themselves in labour. This can only happen in the primal brain. This is also where hypnosis and relaxation take place.

There are certain things that will move a woman from the primal brain back into the neocortex. One of the most obvious is having to answer questions.

A midwife who is asking: 'When did your waters break?' 'How does it feel now?' and 'Can I check your blood pressure?'

A birth partner asking: 'Can I get you anything?' 'Shall I rub your back?'

The neocortex is supposed to be at rest, allowing the primal brain to release birth hormones and make giving birth easy.

What stimulates the neocortex?

- Language – conversation / discussion / questions
- Bright lights
- TV or up-tempo music
- Feeling observed
- Being cold
- Moving location in labour

Nocturnal mammals give birth during the day when there are fewer of their group around. A horse, usually a daytime grazer, will birth at night for the same reason.

Researcher Niles Newton studied mammalian birth in the 1960's. Her findings are just as relevant today. She studied mice giving birth, and there were factors that inhibited or stopped the birth process. These were:

- Placing the labouring mother in an unfamiliar environment (a place where the sights and smells are not what she's accustomed to)
- Moving the mother from one place to another during birth
- Putting the mice in a transparent cage made of glass and observing them

This will sound familiar to you after looking at the section on hormones and birth. We already know that mammals can release oxytocin to begin and continue labour. However if they feel threatened or endangered the emergency hormone is adrenalin.

French obstetrician Michel Odent is a supporter of what he calls unobserved birth. He describes adrenalin and oxytocin as antagonistic hormones (by this we mean they work in opposition with one another), and explains that the basic need of all mammals giving birth is to feel secure. In a wild environment a female cannot give birth as long as there is a possible danger, for example the presence of a predator around. There are no predators in your birth environment, but a human mammal may ***perceive*** the threat.

Considering what we know, is it possible to give the woman the feeling of being unobserved? Can a birth room hold a birth partner and a midwife who do not disturb the pace and rhythm of labour? It is possible, and we have seen it and heard about it. Usually from hypnobirthing partners who are well educated on facilitating the perfect birth environment.

Lisa and Jody's story

I think the hypnobirth techniques made a huge difference to our birth experience, mostly because I felt confident about what was going on inside my body (so didn't feel panicky) and also because Jody had been given lots of tools to help keep us both calm and focused.

When we arrived at the hospital, Jody spent some time setting up the room with aromatherapy oils, coloured LED candles, dimming the lights, laying out blankets and treats and putting my playlist on the sound dock. It felt more like being in a spa than in a hospital room.

I didn't need any pain relief until a couple of hours before our baby was born, as I was able to breathe through the surges calmly. When I started getting the urge to bear down, we requested the birthing pool, which felt amazing and really relaxed me. The whole way through the birth our baby's heartbeat remained strong and healthy and he came out quite happily in the pool, just under 10 hours from when we had first been admitted to Juno.

We had a wonderful birth that was natural, calm and filled with tender moments that, for us as a couple, we will treasure forever. We both feel very strongly that this is because of the training we received in hypnobirth and would definitely recommend the course to anyone who is pregnant. I was able to go home just 4 hours after having our baby, which I'm sure is testament itself to how smooth sailing our birth was.

Also, I do now play the relaxation CD on my iPhone to our baby when he is grizzly (particularly when I change his nappy!) and he always calms right down and listens attentively. The three of us are very happy and grateful for our hypnobirth experience.

There is a growing movement called unassisted birth, or freebirth. These are woman who choose to birth their babies at home without medical support. Sometimes a birth partner or doula is present, and sometimes the woman births completely alone.

Unassisted birth is becoming more and more popular in the UK. The women who plan to birth this way have given it a lot of thought, attended antenatal appointments but choose to birth away from hospitals and medics. Freebirthers believe a woman's body works best when not interfered with. Often women who are attracted to freebirth have experienced previous births where they felt unsupported by the medical team. As midwives we would always prefer to be present and support a woman. We must ask ourselves how can we achieve the level of intimacy, privacy and space for women whilst still offering supportive safe care?

"It is more important that we honour and respect the birthing space of the labouring woman and her most basic, primal needs as a mammal than to use her as a test subject for our own reassurance and education." Grantly Dick-Read 1942.

Section TWO Summary

What Improves the Birth Experience?

- Positive Expectation
- Understanding Cultural Influences
- Understanding and Accepting Birth Rhythms
- Embracing and Celebrating the Rhythms of Womanhood
- Massage
- Water Therapy
- Hot/cold
- The Environment
- Understanding Birth Physiology
- Optimal Positioning of the Pelvis and the Baby
- Relaxation
- Abdominal Breathing
- Feeling Confident
- Support from a Great Birth Partner
- Resting the neocortex

Section THREE

Labour

The Rhythm of Labour

Most antenatal classes will describe labour as first, second and third stage. This sounds clear and easily identifiable. In the maternity world, and the medical world generally, we like structure and numbers. Think about the numbers we define pregnant women by: blood pressure, age, body mass index, glucose tolerance tests, blood results, length of gestation, centimetres dilated, fifths palpable. The list goes on...

You may start to believe you are a set of statistics! Of course numbers can give us important information, and we are not suggesting ignoring them. Nevertheless your cervix has not read the guideline on how women are supposed to dilate. Your baby and body will gestate to a length of time that is appropriate for them and not the textbook. Trying to define labour is like herding cats! You may think you have it, and then something unexpected happens.

Not many births are 'textbook', and when we talk about labour please bear in mind that your body and baby will most likely not conform. Here is a guide to what you might experience.

Pre Labour or Latent Phase

The cervix has been closed for many months, keeping your baby safe inside the uterus, until the time comes for it to open to allow for birth. Remember the cervix is a muscle. You may never have used it before. For any work to take place the muscle wants to prepare, as we would prepare our muscles for any physical exercise. You might stretch a muscle, warm it up, give it time to adjust to working at a different pace. This is exactly what pre labour is doing.

For labour to begin the cervix needs to become softer and thinner and the time this takes can vary considerably. Every woman is different. You may not be aware of it happening. Some women find latent phase surges so mild they do not believe they experienced a latent phase at all. Others may feel the surges so strongly they are convinced this is active labour.

This is an important time, as your body prepares to labour. You are producing the necessary hormones that will begin the birth journey. Your uterus may begin to surge irregularly, trying to figure out which muscle fibres to use for labour. During this time you may be unsure if these are Braxton-Hicks surges or true labour. The cervix starts out firm and long. During pre labour the hormones and the uterine movement cause it to soften, thinning to become pliable enough to stretch over your baby's head. If this is your first labour these changes require more time. By having a slow and steady latent phase you will have time to adjust to labour, as the rhythm and pace of the surges increase.

It is not unusual for women to experience some irregular surges and then a rest. There may be a flurry of activity and then hours of nothing. This is all work that allows your cervix and uterus to become rhythmic. Your body needs time to adjust. Be patient as your body is preparing in small stages. You will move into established labour when your body is ready.

Top Tips for Pre-Labour

- Rest and relax. Try building a nest with bean bags / pillows / duvets so you can be on all fours on the bed / sofa as lying down can be uncomfortable
- Early hospital admission is disruptive. Unless there is a problem, home is where you will be more relaxed
- Use a birth ball. Try rocking on a birthing ball or lean over it
- Hypnobirth breathing and your CD

Contd...

Top Tips for Pre-Labour (contd...)

- Eat and drink well. Fuel your body for the journey ahead
- Go out! Walk the dog; get lunch out, walk in the park. Staying home and watching the clock will make time drag
- Distractions - listening to music, watching TV, try some gardening or bake a cake
- Take a bath. Candles around the bath and nice smells will all feel relaxing
- Massage
- Invite friends over. Ask them to bring lunch!
- Support at this time is important; Birth partners - reassure her and help achieve a calm, tranquil environment
- Keep calm and relaxed so the body can produce the oxytocin needed for a short and easy labour
- Use Rebozo techniques
- Read a script
- Sleep if at all possible. You will probably miss tonight's sleep
- Understand the physiology and know this is normal

The First Stage of Labour

"The first stage of labour is generally recognised as being from the onset of regular uterine contractions and progressive cervical dilatation from 4cms to full dilatation of the cervix" (NICE, 2014)

There will be a time when you move from pre labour into what we call '*established or active labour*'. Established or active labour is usually identified from 4cm dilated.

There are women who reach 6cm dilation and do not realise it. There are others who feel every surge from 1cm. Often you will be at home during this time, and as you have no idea of how many centimetres your cervix is, you can only judge the ***feel*** of your labour.

Surges may become more frequent. Where pre labour may have been irregular, they may now establish a steady pattern.

Counting Surges – Birth partner's role

- Hospitals count surges in 10 minute periods
- Take 10 minutes – let's say from 10am until 10:10am
- How many surges did she experience?
- One surge every 10 minutes is probably still pre labour. As they increase in frequency they are working to soften and open the cervix
- Your midwife will want to know how many surges in 10 minutes

How to cope with a Surge

This is tricky, as every woman is individual and all will experience a surge differently. There may be some general similarities though. Here are some thoughts on the most commonly asked questions about surges.

How long will it last?

An average surge is around a minute and a half. That's 90 seconds. Some will be less, some longer.

What does it feel like?

As the surge begins there will be tightness, like a drum. If you have experienced Braxton-Hicks then it is like this. There is often no sensation at this stage. As it builds the tightness will remain, and sensation will begin. This builds until it reaches the peak. The first part, going up the surge (the bottom section of the surge triangle) can be sensation free. The middle part of the surge will be accompanied by sensation, which may feel more intense. The peak of the surge (top of the triangle) will last an average of 20-30 seconds. As you move over the top of the surge and come down the other side everything eases, releases and relaxes.

What shall I do?

As the surge begins, get comfortable where you are. If you are walking, stop. If you are eating lunch, put down your sandwich! Start your breathing to allow your abdominal muscles to relax and accommodate the tightness. Close your eyes and focus on the breath.

Birth partners: do not talk to her, or allow anyone else to do so. This is incredibly distracting. Do not move her.

As the surge moves up in intensity, the breath will be long and slow to match it. Breathe through it. As it moves upwards to the peak it will require all of your focus. Concentrate on the out breath. The peak is the tricky part, and yet is probably only 30 seconds of the whole surge. Once at the top of the peak the surge begins to release, and you can relax.

When the surge has gone there is no residual sensation. You are completely normal. Continue your walk, your lunch, watching TV or just rest. It was 90 seconds, you can do it!

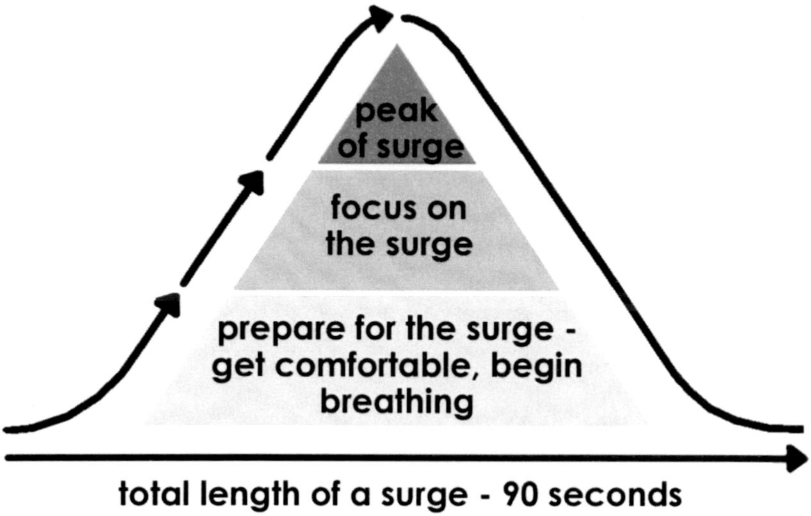

Surge Practice Exercise

- Begin your long slow surge breathing and really focus on the out breath
- Get someone to time your breathing for 30 seconds. This is the peak of the surge and where you will need to focus your breathing the most
- How many breaths did you need to ride the crest of the wave?
- Keep that number of breaths in mind. It will help you focus in labour

Vaginal Examination

During first stage labour the focus of attention tends to be cervix driven. Many women want to know how many centimetres they are dilated. To be able to give you this information the midwife can perform a vaginal examination, also known as a 'V.E.'.

A V.E. is an intimate examination and most women do not welcome the idea. They see it as a necessary evil if they need to know dilatation. Dilatation is never the whole story. Many changes take place during the first stage and the cervix opening is just one of them. It is not an exact science, and although midwives are incredibly skilled, your dilatation can vary from midwife to midwife. The midwives' tools are her fingers, not a tape measure! A V.E. can make or break a woman psychologically. If she feels she has been hours in labour and the resulting V.E. puts her at 2cms dilated she can feel very demoralised.

By contrast an 8cm cervix can spur a woman on as she can see the finishing line.

What you need to know is that your cervix works at its own pace. If it has taken you 10 hours to get to 4cms, that is not a reflection of how long it will take to do another 4cms. Women can go from 4cms to fully open in 20 minutes. So although the information a V.E. gives us is useful, it can also be inaccurate and misleading.

The Essential Guide to V.E.s

- The National Institute for Health and Care Excellence (NICE) state that all women should be offered a V.E. every four hours. Be aware that you can choose to decline the offer of a V.E., or postpone it to a time when you feel ready
- NICE also says "be sure that the examination is necessary and will add important information to the decision making process"
- Should you choose to accept the V.E. it should be performed between surges if possible
- You may need to use your hypnobirth breathing – the more relaxed you are the easier it is
- Midwives can examine women whilst they are in the birth pool
- Once the V.E. is complete make sure you return to an upright comfortable position

Top Tips for First Stage

- Hypnobirth breathing and CD
- Give your body time to establish a rhythm.
- Eat and drink – little and often
- Value the spaces between the surges. This is where you will produce endorphins

Birth partners:

- Is she able to rest, or even sleep, between surges?
- Build a nest, encourage relaxation
- Light touch massage
- 3 step touch breathing if needed
- Being upright, rocking, swaying, birth ball and Rebozo all keep the pelvis open

The Second Stage of Labour

The second stage of labour is defined in two parts: passive second stage and active second stage. From the beginning of labour the cervix has been softening, thinning and opening. It is finally open enough to allow a baby's head to move beyond it. This can be called 10 centimetres although once again we would question the exact measurement. Let's call it fully open!

Your body has been working incredibly hard. There is still work to do, and sometimes it needs to gather its resources. This can result in the surges slowing or even leaving for a while. Midwives call it the 'rest and be thankful' stage! Enjoy this time. Rest, eat, and gather your thoughts. This is passive second stage. This time is not 'counted' in your second stage, and active second stage will commence from the time you feel expulsive surges.

There will come a time when the surges return (if they ever left) and you will feel your baby moving down. This is accompanied by an overwhelming urge to bear down, sometimes referred to as 'pushing'. This is active second stage.

The Big Push?

Much has been debated around the subject of pushing. NICE recommend that women should be guided by their own instinctive urges during second stage. However it has long been a cultural norm for the midwife to direct the woman to 'push'. This has often been accompanied by breath holding and 'pushing into your bottom'. This kind of directed pushing is called the valsalva manoeuvre. Holding the breath at this stage closes the glottis and has many disadvantages. Valsalva pushing reduces oxygen to the woman and the baby. It has been linked with increased perineal trauma and long term effects on bladder and pelvic floor function.

Second stage on TV is usually quick – two pushes and it is all over. In reality active second stage can take anything up to 3 hours for a first time birth. 'Pushing' is a description that suggests that the woman moves her baby significantly with every surge. In fact the baby is 'nudged' down with each surge and this can take a while. When left to instinctively respond to the sensation, women perform a combination of little nudges and longer instinctive 'pushes'. Having a midwife direct this activity is counterproductive. You will work with your body and your baby to a rhythm and pattern that is all your own. During your hypnobirth class your teacher will explain 'J' breathing. This can be used to focus the breath down and into the right place for second stage.

Top Tips for Second Stage

- Know the difference between passive and active second stage
- If you are in passive second stage there should be no suggestion of 'pushing' before your body is ready
- Upright positions will enable birth to be quicker and more comfortable
- Antenatal perineal massage may prevent tearing

Birth partners:

- Encourage 'J' breathing
- Birth partners – ask the staff to refrain from directions- they are not the experts – the birthing woman is!
- A hot compress on the perineum may help to prevent tearing
- Being in a birthing pool may help to prevent tearing

You have an innate ability to birth your baby without direction

The Third Stage of Labour

Once your baby has been birthed there is the placenta to consider. There are two options available to you when considering third stage, a managed third stage or a natural (physiological) third stage. It is important to say that the circumstances surrounding birth will have an impact on your choices.

Active Management of Third Stage

- An injection of oxytocin after birth
- Cord clamping and cutting between 1 and 5 minutes after birth
- Delivery of the placenta by controlled cord traction by the midwife
- Usually takes about 15-30 minutes

Physiological Management of Third Stage

- No injection of oxytocin after birth
- Cord is left unclamped
- Usually takes about 15 minutes – an hour
- The placenta is expelled by the woman-no cord traction

Early cord clamping is defined as clamping in the first 60 seconds after birth. Delayed or deferred cord clamping is more than one minute after birth up until the pulsations have ceased. (World Health Organisation 2015).

The advantages of leaving the cord to pulsate for more than 60 seconds include:

- **Extra 20–30 mg/kg of iron for the newborn which is sufficient for the needs of a newborn for around 3 months. (Royal College of Obstetricians and Gynaecologists 2015)**
- **Continued oxygen supply at a time when the newborn is adjusting to life outside the womb**
- **Stem cell transferral**
- **Placental transfusion provides an additional 80–100ml of blood to the baby (RCOG 2015)**
- **Delayed cord clamping results in better cardiorespiratory transition and more stable blood pressure for baby**

The Cochrane Library produces the best evidence from high quality research. They state:

"Although early cord clamping has been thought to reduce the risk of bleeding after birth (postpartum haemorrhage), this review of 15 randomised trials involving a total of 3911 women and infant pairs showed no significant difference in postpartum haemorrhage rates when early and late cord clamping (generally between one and three minutes) were compared. There were, however, some potentially important advantages of delayed cord clamping in healthy term infants, such as higher birth weight, early haemoglobin concentration, and increased iron reserves up to six months after birth."

The evidence from Cochrane and NICE is clear; deferred cord clamping has many benefits for baby. There is also evidence that the use of oxytocic drugs reduces bleeding after birth.

Your care provider will be observing your blood loss after birth, and ensuring it is within safe limits. If you have chosen a physiological third stage but the blood loss becomes heavy then the oxytocic drug can be administered.

Researcher Sara Wickham writes about third stage. She suggests that the oxytocin drug given after birth quickly constricts the blood vessels, limiting the amount of blood at birth. However once the drug wears off several hours later the body resumes 'normal' blood loss. A physiological third stage results in more blood loss at birth as the uterus is not being artificially constricted. This then slows later. Both types of third stage eventually lose the same amount of blood, at different times.

Many couples feel conflicted by the information available around third stage. Let's assume that birth is very straightforward. We have given birth in a comfortable position, using no medication and baby has arrived healthy. If there has been no need for drugs in labour, we might assume there will be no need for drugs for the third stage. If the labour has experienced a lot of intervention then we cannot expect third stage to progress naturally. In this instance the oxytocic drug is wholly appropriate.

There are women who choose to take a complete physiological approach. This involves not clamping the cord until after the placenta has birthed. There are those who prefer a managed approach. There are others who lotus birth, which involves keeping the baby attached to the placenta after birth until it naturally separates. Our aim is to inform you. Read the evidence, and take advice from your midwife on the day. Look at all the information and birth your placenta the most appropriate way for you.

Alex's story

In order to make my birth space as relaxed as possible, I was encouraged to bring things which would make me comfortable. Examples included a playlist, food and drink and objects to support me during birth. I therefore readied myself with over 76 hours of music, 3 multipacks of Ribena and 3 boxes of Tracker bars; I was clearly expecting a long haul! Syrie, my birth partner, also suggested more practical items which she found useful during her own labours and supported an active birth, such as a giant bean bag and hot water bottles.

Completely subconsciously, I found myself migrating to a more intimate space as had been described during my hypnobirthing classes. I largely stayed there for about 5 hours, after which time the surges intensified and I decided it was time to head back to hospital.

Top Tips for Third Stage

- As with labour, do your research. Look at the differences between a managed and natural third stage and write your preferences in your birth plan
- Remain flexible. It may be that labour circumstances dictate third stage
- If you are choosing a managed third stage consider requesting the full 5 minutes of delayed cord clamping
- Decide who cuts the cord. Do not worry about this part. The staff will be there to guide you. Birth partners-there is no shame if you cannot think of anything worse!
- Just like labour, third stage is susceptible to hormones. Oxytocin must remain high. Keep baby skin to skin. Stay warm. Keep the environment quiet, calm and the lights dim
- Putting your baby to the breast will help to stimulate oxytocin, producing the surges needed for placental separation
- Gravity often helps birth a placenta
- After birth your midwife will check the placenta. If you are interested she/he can explain the placenta and show it to you. Some couples keep it to bury in the garden. Some women like to eat the placenta postnatally. It is said to rebalance hormones and aid recovery. There is little research into this but you can find more information at www.placentanetwork.com

Caesarean Birth and Hypnobirth

For some women the most appropriate way to give birth is by caesarean birth. Many couples have used the hypnobirth techniques to prepare for a calm gentle birth. Once a caesarean has been decided, many women feel they have no choice or control. The surgery itself needs to be performed safely and there are certain procedures to be followed. However it is wise to talk with your doctor and midwife beforehand, ask questions and work on a way to achieve your calm gentle birth.

The microbiome and birth

Emerging research shows that bacteria are absolutely vital for human health, and imbalances in the human microbiome significantly contribute to chronic non-transmissible diseases. The microbiome is gut bacteria that is cultured during the vaginal birth process. The baby is 'seeded' as it passes through the birth canal. Babies born by caesarean birth have a third less bacteria variety than babies born vaginally. This can have an impact on long term health. A documentary called Microbirth (www.microbirth.com) explains how women experiencing a caesarean birth can reproduce the optimum gut flora. This is called 're-seeding'.

At least an hour before birth the mother inserts a sterile gauze that has been soaked in normal saline into the vaginal birth canal. The gauze needs to be folded, like a tampon, with lots of surface area. This will culture the trillions of bacteria that are usually passed to the baby during birth.

The sterile gauze is removed just before birth and kept in a sterile container. Once the baby is birthed the gauze is used to wipe the baby's face, nose, mouth and rest of the body (the parents can do this, or the midwife).

"As the fetus grows in the womb, it develops in a near-sterile environment relying on its mother for protection. But when the baby emerges, it is entering a world of bacteria, some of which are bad (pathogens) but some of which are good.

In the weeks and days leading up to birth, specific species of good bacteria are migrating to key locations in the mother's body and are transferred to the baby during and immediately after birth via the birth canal, immediate skin-to-skin contact and breastfeeding. The role of these good bacteria is to train the baby's human cells to distinguish between what is "friend" and what is "foe" so that its immune system can fight off attack from pathogens. This process kickstarts the baby's immune system, and helps to protect the infant from disease for its entire lifetime.

However, with interventions like the use of synthetic oxytocin, antibiotics, C-section and formula feeding, this microbial transfer from the mother to baby is interfered with or bypassed completely. For babies that enter the world by C-section, their first contact could be with bacteria that are resident in hospitals and from strangers, i.e. not with the special cocktail of bacteria from the mother.

The latest scientific research is now starting to indicate that if the baby is not properly seeded with the mother's own bacteria at birth, then the baby's microbiome, in the words of Rodney R Dietert, Professor of Immunotoxicology at Cornell University, is left "incomplete". Consequently, that baby's immune system may never develop to its full potential, leaving that infant with an increased risk of developing one or more serious diseases later in life".

Toni Harman- Microbirth.

Hypnobirth Techniques for Caesarean Birth

- Eye opening and closing script – practice this at home. The birth partner will find it easy to count and initiate relaxation using this
- Shoulder anchor – easy to reach and very effective
- Counting and breathing technique
- Golden thread, ice cube and eye of the storm are all short enough to use as surgery begins

Top Tips for Caesarean Birth

- Before the birth there will be a wait. Often a planned caesarean takes preparation time. Use the surge breathing techniques to stay calm and relaxed
- Birth partners can use 3 step touch breathing during this time
- Play the hypnobirth CD in the wait before birth, and ask the staff to play it for you in theatre
- Use a tissue and place a drop of your favourite relaxing aromatherapy oil on it. (The one you have used to relax to at home is best). Give it to the birth partner to put into the pocket of their scrubs. This can be used during the birth – a quick sniff will be a trigger for relaxation.

Contd....

Contd....

- If you wish you can ask for the drape to be lowered at the moment of birth. You will not see any of the surgery, but the doctor can lift baby and you will be able to see those first moments
- If you do not know the sex of the baby and wish to discover it for yourselves remember to say so. The drape lowering moment may be ideal for this
- Can your doctor allow the cord to pulsate for a little while? Ask. Even 30 seconds longer is beneficial to your baby
- Skin to skin contact with you should be initiated immediately after birth. If this is not possible for some reason then skin to skin with the birth partner
- Ask for baby to be weighed after prolonged skin to skin and with you in the room. Remember to ask for baby to be placed tummy down in the scales. This is an instinctive fetal position for baby and causes less distress
- If you would like vitamin K for your baby why not ask for it to be administered whilst baby is skin to skin or breastfeeding? This limits time spent away from baby and softens the moment of injection for the baby
- Take a camera and record the moments after birth. They will be precious
- Consider taking probiotics postnatally

Section FOUR

Upright Birth

Upright Birth

When you visualise giving birth to your baby, is there a bed involved? Think about birth portrayed on TV. Mostly we see bed birth. Historically women have been birthing in bed for many years. It may have something to do with hospital birth. If you are in a hospital then you are a patient. If you are a patient then you must be sick, and in bed. The maternity setting is the only place where you are in a hospital yet fit and well.

There has been much written about bed birth, and what we mean by bed birth is lying down. It can also be called the supine position. What we know is that lying on your back for labour has many disadvantages. The term 'active birth' was coined by Janet Balaskas in the 1970s. Before this all women were expected to birth on their backs in bed. The mammalian pelvis is designed for upright birth. When the baby descends through the pelvis the sacrum and coccyx are able to move back, gaining the woman **28% more space.** It makes complete sense that to move a baby down and through the pelvis the birth must involve the advantage of gravity.

Remaining upright can also have an effect on pain in labour: a study published in 2003 confirmed a labouring woman's lower back pain is worse when she is lying down (Adachi, Shimada, & Usai, 2003).

Regular rhythmic movement in labour helps women cope with the surges. Women instinctively move, sway and rock to ease pressure. The baby is able to position himself optimally if the pelvis is upright and open.

What's wrong with this picture? **The same thing that's wrong with this one!**

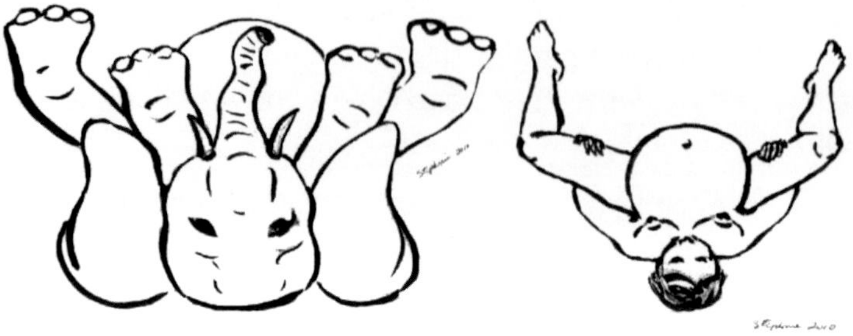

Imagine trying to restrict an elephant to give birth on her back...

It would probably require drugs and might lead to surgery

Imagine trying to restrict a woman to give birth on her back...

It would probably require drugs and might lead to surgery

[Reproduced with kind permission of Stephanie Larson founder of Dancing for Birth™ www.dancingforbirth.com]

A Cochrane review in 2009 confirms that women experience shorter labours when upright and were less likely to need epidural analgesia. You will feel in control and empowered when you are mobile and active in labour.

Upright Birth vs Bed Birth

Upright	***Lying down***
Space in pelvis increased by 28%	Decreased pelvic space
Deep abdominal breathing possible	Shallow chest breathing
Freedom of movement helps pain	Being immobile increases pain
Less likely to experience perineal tear	More likely to tear
Increased oxygen for baby	Decreased oxygen for baby
Quicker birth	Slower birth
More likely to give birth naturally	More likely to need assisted birth
Baby's head dilates cervix	Pressure off cervix results in slow dilatation
Less likely to need epidural	More likely to need epidural

The Challenges of Upright Birth

Many maternity units have embraced the active birth philosophy. They will fully support your expectations of birth off the bed. The challenge can often be the environment and equipment. Environment creates expectation. Many birth rooms still contain beds. Many women when shown into a birth room with a bed in the centre will go and get on it.

This is without being asked, as the culture of a hospital is such that women expect to be on a bed. If this is the dominant bit of equipment when you walk into the room then you have to start thinking of rearranging the room. Please bear in mind the importance of the environment, and how many hours you may spend in this room. It is ***your*** birth room, and should be ***made*** to work for you. This will help:

- Push the bed to the side of the room. It's on wheels!
- If the bed has a function to move it into a chair position then do so

Ask for:

- A floor mat
- A beanbag
- A birth ball
- A birthing stool
- Use a Rebozo (bring your own)

Ask your midwife if your hospital has all of these available.

If labour requires continuous fetal monitoring this can be done with you sitting next to the monitor on a birth ball, or standing. Ask if the hospital use telemetry. This is wireless monitoring which does not restrict movement. It can also be waterproof for a pool birth.

Birth off the bed will benefit you and your baby. Move and work with your instincts. If this means some time on the bed then so be it. This is your labour. However the positions you choose should never be influenced by the convenience of others. Midwives are incredibly adaptable, and will be more than happy to listen to your baby in whatever position you choose.

Encouraging your baby into the best position for birth

During pregnancy your baby will settle into the space within your pelvis, and as he grows you may be able to feel which position the baby favours. Most babies want to be head down. The head is the heaviest part of your baby, and acts to 'anchor' baby in the pelvis. Some babies will prefer to be bottom down, known as breech. Whichever part of your baby is in the pelvis is known as the 'presenting part'.

As the baby is lying in water, the spine of the baby will rotate, facing toward the maternal abdomen, or the maternal spine. The baby positioned towards the mother's abdomen is known as occipito-anterior (OA) or ANTERIOR for short.

The baby positioned towards the mother's spine is known as occipito-posterior (OP) or POSTERIOR for short.

Anterior Position

The OA or anterior position is the most effective way for your baby to journey through the pelvis. However the baby can move towards the left or right side of the abdomen, and this makes a difference.

The uterus has a natural curve on the left side. If the baby maximises this position and settles into the curve, the baby will achieve head flexion. This means that the baby's chin will tuck nicely into her chest, allowing the 'presenting part', the top of the head, to be the smallest diameter and to fit snugly over the cervix. This helps it to dilate and open effectively.

If the baby settles to the right of the uterus there is less curve and therefore less head flexion. Labour can be slower.

Posterior Position

When the baby adopts an OP or posterior position the spine of the baby is less curved than the anterior positioned baby. The head is less flexed, meaning that the presenting part of the head is larger. This can encourage the baby to rotate into the anterior position during labour, but can make labour slower. It may affect the pattern of the labour, resulting in irregular surges. It is also important to bear in mind that this position may not affect labour at all and babies can be born in the posterior position. It is a good idea to ask your midwife which position your baby is in, and begin to think about optimal fetal positioning.

Optimal Fetal Positioning

Optimal fetal positioning (OFP) is a term introduced by Jean Sutton and Pauline Scott in 1996. They predicted more babies were assuming the OP position due to women's lifestyle. We tend to spend time sitting on the sofa or reclining in a chair with our bottom lower than the knees. This encourages our babies to rotate around towards the spine. Car seats are another culprit and encourage the OP position.

Your baby can only access the space available within the pelvis. Gail Tully (spinningbabies.com) discusses the importance of balance within the pelvis. She argues that the ligaments, muscles and fascia of the uterus can influence the position of the baby. When they are tight, the baby has no alternative but to settle into the space available. There are many ways to regain balance within the pelvis, and the Spinning Babies website is a great source of information. Use the top tips to begin to encourage your baby into his or her best birth position.

Top Tips for Optimal Fetal Positioning

- Use a birth ball to align the pelvis. Once sitting on it your knees should be lower than your hips
- Use it to watch TV instead of your sofa
- Sit facing the back of a chair 'cowboy style'. This will tilt your pelvis forward. (This position may not be suitable if you experience pelvic girdle pain)
- Put a wedge cushion under your bottom when driving
- Use a beanbag or your birth ball, kneel on the floor and rest over it. Remember to place cushions under your knees. You can also adapt this by using your birth ball on your sofa and kneeling over it
- If you sit at work use a wedge or a pillow to under your bottom. You should be sitting on your tuberosities (the bony part of your bum) not your sacrum
- Do not cross your legs. This reduces the space at the front of the pelvis and opens it up at the back. For good positioning, the baby needs to have lots of space at the front
- Swimming puts your baby into a great position
- Exercises done on all fours can help - wiggling your hips from side to side, or arching your back like a cat, followed by levelling the spine

Contd....

- Standing and rotating the hips encourages movement. Think belly dancing! Circle one way, then the other. Try a figure of eight.
- If you experience practice surges try to use these positions to encourage baby rotation
- Avoid deep squatting until you know the baby is in the best position. Deep squats encourage the baby to move down – great if the position is OA
- Use the rebozo techniques you have learnt in class

Section FIVE

Hypnotherapy Techniques Explained

Induction of Hypnosis

In clinical hypnotherapy a state of hypnosis is induced in many different ways depending on the outcome required by the client, although initially we would normally use relaxation until the client is comfortable with the whole process. In hypnobirth, because our goal is deep relaxation and calm, it makes sense to use relaxation for the induction.

Before I became a hypnotherapist I had a very stressful career in the corporate world and found it very difficult to switch off and relax. But during my training, as I practiced hypnotherapy techniques, including self hypnosis, I became better and better at relaxation. Now, even on stressful days, and let's face it we all have them, all I need to do is take a couple of deep breaths and let go. This means that as you practice, you will find that you become relaxed more and more easily.

Self Hypnosis

Self hypnosis is simply when you use the techniques that you have learned in class and use them effectively on your own. Because hypnosis is a natural state of being, we don't need anyone else to put us into that state. Once you know what you are doing you can easily do it for yourself, although sometimes it's nice to have someone else to prompt, encourage or guide us.

Triggers and Anchors

Triggers are very powerful. When we want to change an unwanted behaviour it is important to identify the actions that trigger this particular habit. For smokers there are lots of common triggers, e.g. when the telephone rings; after a meal; or with a glass of wine. So when breaking a habit such as smoking; identifying the triggers and changing them in even a small way can help the process. I overheard a conversation recently between a young woman who is in the process of becoming a non-smoker and a man who has been a non-smoker for several years now.

She said "I'm doing really well, except when I'm at work. If someone else goes outside for a cigarette, I really want to go with them. But I don't smoke at all when I'm at home – I don't even think about it."

He responded: "I really struggled when I used to go out to the pub for a drink. So I stopped going for a while until I had cracked it, and now I can have a beer without wanting a cigarette, it's great!"

We know that stress and anxiety are unwanted during labour because they can lead to the Stress/Tension/Pain cycle. We also want to avoid stress and anxiety during pregnancy in order to create a calm environment for the baby to develop. This is why it is essential to avoid listening to negative birth stories, whether that's from family and friends or television soaps, dramas or documentaries. It is also why it is important to practice your relaxation every day to counteract the normal day-to-day stresses.

Triggers can also be used in a positive way; to remind us to do a task. For example, every time you are stopped by a red light you can remember to do your pelvic floor exercise, or to take some abdominal breaths to increase the flow of oxygen and relax your body and mind.

Start to create triggers to remind you of the positive techniques that you want to adopt and then practice them every day until they become a habit. This will allow you both to feel confident during labour, so that mums can stay 'in the zone' and dads or birthing partners know what to do without pulling her back into the neocortex.

Anchors are physical cues to a feeling of relaxation or to strengthen a particular suggestion. They are simple and easy to use. The shoulder anchor is used to deepen relaxation. The birth partner will use a gentle downward pressure on the shoulder that instantly triggers this feeling of deep relaxation in the woman.

Matching and Pacing

Matching and pacing is a technique that we can use to take someone else from one state into a different state. First you must match the state that they are in and then gradually move into the state that you would like them to be in. Let's look at some examples:

I was recently in a hotel reception where a customer was extremely unhappy with the service he had received. The receptionist said something that was clearly the final straw and the man exploded into angry shouting which ended with the manager being called. The customer continued to shout his displeasure and at first the manager also spoke in quite a loud voice. Very quickly the manager slowed the pace of his speech and reduced the volume and within a short space of time the angry customer began to calm. He then apologised for his outburst and was willing to listen to the manager who did his best to rectify the problem.

Another wonderful example of using matching and pacing to good effect was a story told to me by a midwife. She was caring for a woman whose labour was going quite slowly and it was outside the time frame set by the hospital. A doctor came into the room demanding to know why this woman hadn't already been put on a drip. He was rather loud and brusque and was interrupting the calm relaxation in the room.

The midwife smiled at the doctor and then turned to the women and began to talk to her is a calm voice, suggesting that she take some long slow breaths, that she notice herself become more and more calm. She continued in this way for several minutes during which time the doctor's hands had dropped to his sides, his breathing had slowed and his state of mind had changed. He then said that perhaps she could be left a little longer as all seemed to be well and he left the room. The woman went on to birth her baby naturally.

We can see from this that it is possible to influence others indirectly with calm breathing and gentle words.

On another occasion a father reported to me that a doctor had come into their room with much the same attitude and when asked if he had read their birth plan, the doctor answered that he had not. The dad suggested that he go and read it and come back again later. The doctor left the room and didn't return. They went on to have a calm birth even though it had been rather slow.

The three-step touch breathing is excellent for bringing the mother from a moment of anxiety, or even panic, back into the zone. One of the important things to remember when you are using this technique is to match her breathing to begin with and then to help her to slow down.

As you rest your hand on her chest breathe with her. After only a breath or two, begin to slow your breathing and move your hand into the second position. Breathe so that she can hear you, and make it even slower as you move into the third position. You will find that as she focuses on your hand, noticing the warmth, she will slow her breathing with you and can become wonderfully calm.

This matching and pacing technique can be used in many situations. There may be times when you find yourselves doing it instinctively. Perhaps you will be doing some relaxing massage during the early stages of labour and will notice your breathing becoming synchronised.

Deepeners

Deepeners are exactly what they sound! They are used to deepen relaxation. The more relaxed you become the further you move from engaging your neocortex which allows you to use your instincts to great effect.

As well as the Staircase Deepener, we also use deepeners within the scripts; they are simple suggestions to go deeper into relaxation. The more you embrace the suggestions and let yourself go, the more effective they will be. Some days it's easier than others to let go, so just practice and know that each time you practice you will strengthen the habit to become more and more relaxed.

Using Scripts

You should become familiar with the scripts very quickly, whether you're listening to the CD or your birth partner reads them to you.

You may decide that you'd like to be creative with the scripts and techniques, so let's break down a typical script.

Induction – the progressive relaxation that takes you into hypnosis

Deepener – to take you further and further into relaxation

Visualisation – to take you on a relaxing journey, perhaps to create a calm safe space to imagine during labour

Affirmations – these can be included in this section, just as they are on the CD

Emerge from hypnosis – this will bring you from deep hypnosis back to fully conscious awareness. Of course, during hypnobirth we want you to stay in a relaxed state, so we would simply suggest that you stay in that lovely feeling of relaxation for as long as you want. You might even fall asleep.

Creating your own script

So now that you know the components of a script you can begin to adapt them and create your own. Think about the words and phrases that you particularly like, e.g.

- Relax, relax, relax
- Confident, powerful and strong
- Release, relax, let go
- Down and down and down
- Breathing in, and breathing out, breathing in, and breathing out, breathing in, and breathing out

- Soft, loose, relaxed
- Calm, quiet and open
- Peaceful, instinctive and happy

Mothers often tell us how a particular word or group of words became a mantra though her surges.

Do you respond to counting? With the out breath.... 5, 4, 3, 2, 1. If this works for you then add it into your script.

In the CD we have included a beach visualisation; we want you to find your own calm, safe space in nature. This could be real, a memory or imagined. It is important you describe it to your birth partner as they will be describing it in the script.

- It may be a beach from a holiday you have experienced. You might hear the waves as they break on the shore. Can you smell the sea air? Can you feel warm sun on your face? Are you lying on warm soft sand? Can you feel your body sinking into relaxation as you feel the warm sand beneath you?

- Is it woodland, where you can hear birdsong or the rustle of leaves being blown by a gentle breeze? Can you smell flowers, the earthy woody smell of trees? Is there dappled sunlight?

- Are you sitting in a meadow of wild flowers? Can you hear the breeze lightly moving the long grass? Perhaps you can smell freshly cut grass

- Are you on a river bank? Can you hear the sound of water gurgling around you? Are there dragonflies lightly skimming the river? Maybe you hear the occasional fish break the surface of the water, sending soothing ripples across the surface

- You could be lying in a deep, warm sweet smelling bubble bath. The temperature is perfect. Your body feels supported by the warm water. Maybe there are scented candles around your bath?

- Your calm place could be a room. Imagine the furnishings, what is there to relax on? How does the room make you feel? Safe? Relaxed? Sleepy?

So you can see that although we started with one idea, it became something else. That's the beauty of hypnosis and visualisation – you can allow your thoughts to take you wherever they want; you are limited only by your own creativity.

Script Building Template

Here is a script building template to create a script that's just right for you... *[fill in the blanks]* *Instructions are in brackets{ }*

Birth Partners: start reading here...

Sit back and relax. Close your eyes. Take a breath in through the nose. As you breathe out

[Your 3 words]..

And again with the next out breath

[Your 3 words]..

Allow your breath to slow and deepen, slow and deepen, slow and deepen

When you breathe out next I will count from 5 down to 1. With each number down you can allow your body to release, relax, just let go

{Watch for her to take a breath IN....... And as she breathes out count}

5... 4... 3... 2... 1 ... RELAX

5... 4... 3... 2... 1 ... RELAX

5... 4... 3... 2... 1 ... RELAX

As you begin to relax deeper and deeper, imagine yourself in your calm place

Imagine the *[...]*

Find somewhere to sit or lie down comfortably. Make the temperature just right for you

Maybe you can hear *[...]*

Maybe you can smell *[..]*

Allow your body to relax in this special place....

[Your 3 words]..

As you continue to go deeper and deeper, imagine a colour. This is your calm colour of relaxation. Breathe the colour in; allow it to fill your mind, soothing you, bringing with it a deep sense of wellbeing.

This colour can wash over you like a wave from the top of your head, down into your shoulders which loosen and relax.

The calming colour moves down your arms, down into your upper arms, down your lower arms, into your hands which soften and relax.

Allow the colour to move down the rest of your body, your torso, your stomach and down into your legs. Finally you feel the colour in your feet. Feel the weight of your feet as your body lets go of all tension.

[Your 3 words]..

In a moment you will feel my hand on your ....

When you feel the touch of my hand you will double your relaxation, deeply relaxed now.

{Place hand for touch}

Every time you feel my hand here, your breathing will slow down, your body will relax and you can go even deeper and deeper into relaxation than the last time.

[Your 3 words]..

Exercise: Use the template and have fun creating your own favourites...

Additional Scripts

Here are two deep relaxation scripts that are really simple and easy to use and very popular. Practice them with your birth partner who may want to read them through first. ***[Instructions are in brackets]***.

Deep Relaxation

[Start the music and begin script – very slowly...]

So, if you haven't already, make yourself comfortable and close your eyes and settle back, and begin to take some nice deep breaths. Practicing your lovely relaxing breathing... Breathe in deeply ... just so that you're comfortable and then exhale slowly ... very slowly. Allow yourself to become calm and relaxed and continue to breathe in ...... and ... out........ In ..... and .out.....

I'm going to count from 25 down to 1 and when I get to 1 you will feel more relaxed than you've ever felt before. If you want to you can imagine yourself in a lift, make it really comfortable, just right for you. The right size, nice and cozy; the right temperature, maybe you have a comfy sofa to relax on. And as you relax you can see the numbers of the floors as we go down from 25 to 1. As you become more and more relaxed you may not even notice the numbers, all you'll notice is the sound of my voice and how good you feel...

Contd....

[This next part should be read as slowly as possible with long pauses]

So....

25 – nice and comfortable, breathing in ..... and out .... softly ...... and gently ***[pause]***

24 – allowing yourself to go deeper ...... and deeper into relaxation ***[pause]***

23 – more ... and more relaxed ***[pause]***

22 – deeper .... and deeper ***[pause]***

21 – feeling your body drifting down...... further ...... and further ***[remember to pause after each number, getting slower and slower]***

20 – down .... and down

19 – peace ... and calm .... and relaxation

18 – relax ..... relax .... relax

17 – release .... relax .... just let go

16 – deeper .... and deeper

In a moment I'm going to put my hand on your shoulder, and as I press gently downwards, you can allow yourself to feel five times more relaxed than you feel right now.

Contd....

And every time I touch your shoulder, or any part of you, you can allow yourself to feel five times more relaxed. More relaxed than you've ever been...

[Then as she breathes out you put your hand on her shoulder, apply a gentle downward pressure that feels soft and reassuring as you continue to count. Apply pressure on the out breathe and release on the in breath.]

15 – relax ..... relax ..... relax ..... ***[read even slower now]***

14 – deeper ..... and deeper

13 – down ..... and down

[Remove your hand for a moment]

12 – peace .... calm .... relaxation

11 – release .... relax .... just let go

10 – safe ..... calm .... and comfortable. More and more relaxed

In a moment I'm going to touch your shoulder again, and as I do you can go five times deeper, more and more relaxed.

[Touch and release – as before]

9 – deeper ..... and deeper

Contd....

8 – down ..... and down

7 – peace .... calm .... relaxation

[Remove your hand for a moment]

6 – release .... relax .... just let go

5 – down ..... and down

4 – deeper .... and deeper

In a moment I'm going to touch your shoulder again, and as I do you can go five times deeper still, more relaxed than you've ever been.

[Touch and release – as before]

3 – relax ...... relax ...... relax

2 – down ...... and down

and 1 – safe ..... calm .... and comfortable. More and more relaxed

Now you can stay in this feeling of relaxation as long as you want. Resting in this space where time means nothing – an hour seems like a minute. A minute is just a blink. Rest in this space, relax, relax, relax.

Contd....

[If it's bedtime, read this paragraph] Now allow yourself to drift into a beautiful peaceful night's sleep.

[Otherwise, read this paragraph] In a moment it will be time to come back into the room, feeling confident and relaxed, knowing that each time you do this you will find it easier and easier to relax and you will feel more and more confident about the birth of our/your baby. So you can begin by moving your fingers and toes and very gently, in your own time you can open your eyes, feeling great.

Birth partner – every time you practice this script you can read it more and more slowly, make the pauses longer as you go through the script.

Now try the Touch Relaxation so that you can discover how deeply relaxed you can become. Both of these scripts use touch which prepares you to feel calm and relaxed whenever anyone touches you during labour.

You won't have time to practice these in class, so remember to practice them regularly and they will soon become favourites!

Touch Relaxation

Allow your breath to slow and deepen. Slow and deepen.

Breathing in and breathing out. Breathing in and breathing out.

Your body responds to your breath by softening and relaxing. Release, relax, just let go.

You can begin to notice the sounds around you. The noises in the room, the sounds outside the room. Focus on any external sounds and recognise that these sounds make you feel more and more relaxed. You remain relaxed and peaceful whenever you hear noise.

If anyone moves you or touches you, you can double your relaxation.

Focus your attention on your head. In a moment you will feel the warm pressure of my hands on your head.

[Place your hands on her head]

Feel your head and scalp begin to release and relax with the touch. Allow your breathing to slow and deepen. Put your awareness where you feel the touch. Feel the warmth of the touch, and slow your breath. Your mind relaxes...... Thoughts may wander in.....allow them to wander out again. Release any tension in your head and scalp as you breathe softly and slowly, allowing your mind to calm and clear.

In a moment you will feel a calming hand on your forehead.

[Place one hand on her forehead; place the other hand on the base of her skull]

Contd....

This is a touch you can relax into. Feel the warmth and pressure of both hands on your head, and allow it to soothe and calm your mind. Slow and deepen your breath. Allow all tension to release, relax, just let go. This is the peace and calm you can experience in labour. This touch will calm your mind and relax your body whenever you feel it. Let go of all tension. Put your trust in your ability to relax.

In a moment you will feel the touch move to your shoulders.

[Place both hands on her shoulders]

Notice the warmth and relaxation that the pressure creates in your shoulders. Breathing in, and breathing out. Breathing in, and breathing out. As you focus on your long slow out breath, notice how relaxed your shoulders can become. Allow them to sink gently into the frame of your body. Heavy. Relaxed. Just let go.

As you continue to relax into the touch, allow the relaxation to travel like a wave along and down your arms..... Down into your upper arms which relax and loosen........ down into your elbows which soften........ Down into your lower arms which become loose and limp.

Allow this relaxation to move down into your hands which feel heavy and limp. Feel them become warm, heavy. They may begin to tingle. Your hands feel large. Too heavy to move.

In a moment you can feel your hands being touched. As you feel this touch, you can double and deepen your relaxation. Any noises you hear will make your relaxation deeper and deeper. More and more relaxed.

Contd....

[Begin stroking her hand]

Focus on the feeling in your hands. Breathe into it. Allow your hands to soften and relax, loose and limp. Trust that every time you experience this touch it will allow you to deepen your relaxation, just as you will when you give birth to your baby. Your breathing is slow and steady. Your body is calm and relaxed.

In a moment you will feel a hand on your abdomen. Any movement or sounds can deepen your relaxation.

As you feel the pressure of touch on your abdomen, slow and deepen your breath. Allow your out breath to meet the warmth of my hand. Breathe into my hand. Slow and steady. Each long slow breath relaxes you further and further.

Know that you are in control of your body. Allow my touch to help you to decide how relaxed you can be in labour. Each touch can bring you deeper and deeper into calm relaxation. As your body softens and opens, allowing your baby to be born calmly, gently and comfortably, just as you intend.

Each time you practice this you will go quicker and deeper into calm relaxation. And on the day of your birth you will find it easy to allow your body to soften and open, to release and let go.

In a moment it will be time to come back into the room, feeling confident and relaxed. So you can begin by moving your fingers and toes and very gently, in your own time you can open your eyes, feeling great.

Three Step Touch Breathing

Birth partner: begin with your hand lightly resting on her chest

Mummy: close your eyes. Focus on where your partner's hand is resting and breathe into the hand

Birth partner: move your hand to the top of her abdomen, resting on the top of the bump, just under the breastbone. Leave your hand here for 3 breaths

Mummy: focus on the hand. Feel the pressure and warmth. Breathe into the hand

Birth partner: move your hand to the bottom of her abdomen, below the belly button. Check the pressure with her. Leave your hand here for 5 breaths

Mummy: focus on the hand. Feel the pressure and warmth. Breathe into the hand. Try to push the hand away with your out breath

Counting and Breathing

Birth Partner Practice

Your aim is to physically relax your body on one out breath

Take the breath in through your nose. As you breathe out through your mouth visualise the sections of the body

5 – Relax your head and face

4 – Relax your shoulders and chest

3 – Relax your stomach

2 – Relax your thighs

1 – Relax your calves and feet

Repeat 3 times

Letting Go of Anxiety

Typically the people who choose hypnobirth fall into two groups: those who have heard how great it is from their family, friends or their midwife; and those who are feeling anxious and are looking for something to help them feel more confident. In this section we are going to look at two simple techniques you can use to reduce anxiety.

Changing Your Perspective

It's not an incident that causes us a problem, but how we feel about it. Two people can have a very similar experience and one person can feel okay about it, whilst the other may feel upset, anxious or even traumatised by it.

The first technique is in two parts. Part one is done at home between the second and third session. You and your birth partner will take a little to time to think about all the things that make you anxious. Write them down and rate them from 1 to 5 (1 is insignificant and 5 is making you very anxious).

Once you have both created your own list, sit down together and discuss everything that is on the list. We have found that when couples do this they can very often sort out a lot of things that are making them a bit anxious.

For example I was working with a couple and the mum was worrying about who would look after her toddler Charlie, when she went into labour. Her mother lived quite a long way away and her mother-in-law was older and although she had offered to look after her grandson, he had never stayed with her overnight. As they discussed this together, the dad immediately phoned his mother and asked whether they could organise a sleep-over for Charlie. It took a couple of goes, but within a short time Charlie was happy to spend the night with Granny, and so the problem was resolved because they had discussed it and found a great solution.

Now this may seem an obvious thing to do, but sometimes these small anxieties are simply in the back of our minds and we plan to sort them out later. This exercise will help you identify and resolve the practical issues early on, which will mean that you can relax and enjoy your pregnancy.

Some anxieties are less practical and can fall into the "What if..." camp; these thoughts may have come about because of a previous experience of your own or someone else's. This is why the hypnobirth course works to distance you from negative stories from the media, friends and family, and this technique will help you to release or change any thoughts that are already making you anxious.

You will identify the anxiety that you want to release in part one, and in part two we use a visualisation exercise to create some distance from the thought and then to change your perspective. If your anxieties persist and you feel that you would like additional support, talk to your hypnobirth teacher, or your own midwife, who will be able to help you find further professional help.

Imagine a Hug!

Here is another very simple technique that you can use when you feel stressed or anxious which emulates the behaviour of a young child. When a child feels stressed or anxious she will turn to her primary caregiver, holding up her arms, sometimes crying, looking to be soothed and comforted. Now as adults we don't necessarily behave in this way, perhaps the person we would turn to for a hug is unavailable at that moment. However, you can find comfort from the thought of a hug from that person or the memory of someone who gave you loving support or protection. This can create the same feelings for security and comfort as the actual event did.

We have looked at the power of language and of the mind; this is another simple example of the amazing resources that you already possess that you can tap into with imagery, memory and imagination.

Combine this with your relaxation breathing and you are already creating your own toolkit of confidence and power.

Section SIX

Getting Ready for Birth

Top Tips for Birth Partners

- Learn the relaxation techniques with your partner. The breathing will be second nature to her by the time birth comes. However there will always be the surge that takes her breath away. YOU know how to bring it back

  Try the 3 step touch breathing and practice lots.

- Plan the birth together, and write it down. You will be the spokesperson on the day and convey the wishes of your partner

- Know which scripts she prefers and pack them

- Do you have the birth kit ready? Consider a play list of music for labour. Include the hypnobirth CD. Can you put it onto a phone or iPod? Lip balm, flannels and hair bands all become really important! Massage oils? Cold water spray for her face? Aromatherapy oils? TENS machine? Rebozo? Have you thought about nice food and drink to take with you?

- Pack the birth bag yourself. When you want the cold flannel, the lip balm or some spare pants you will be able to lay your hands on them without turning everything out of the bag

- Help your partner to prepare physically for the birth ahead. Consider Aquanatal classes or pregnancy yoga classes. Buy a birth ball and encourage her to use it for sitting on in the evening. This will encourage the baby into a great position and gently stretch the mum's thighs in preparation for birth. Remind her to do pelvic floor exercises and perineal massage

- Support the hypnobirth language. Encourage her to use the affirmations

- In early labour keep things normal. Take her out for a walk/lunch. Run her a bath, watch her favourite DVDs (funny ones are great) play music, massage her

- If you move from home to a birthing unit, build her a nest once you get there. Women often feel unsettled by the move

- Birth room environment – dim the lights – have you considered LED candles? Play her music; make the room smell nice using aromatherapy oils. Move the bed if it is in the middle of the room. Make her a nest using bean bags, pillows and blankets. Put her own pillow/blanket over the bed. Is there a birth ball? A birthing stool? Do you have a floor mat for birth positions? Ask the midwife for these. Bring out nice food and drink, and relax!

- Is the hypnobirth room sign up?

- In labour, help her to find her own rhythm and flow. Often women want to move, rock or sway. Help her to change position and suggest new ones. Use your Rebozo. Think about the resting time between the surges, and how you can make her comfortable

- Look after your own needs. Birth takes stamina for all involved. Have a man bag! A change of clothes (hospitals are often hot) flip flops, your own food and drink and toiletries to enable you to freshen up

- Create a calm and loving environment. If/when there is nothing to be done, just be there silently for her

- Discuss the birth plan with the midwife

The Comfort Birth Kit

- Heat – small hot water bottle
- Cold – frozen gel pack or a small bottle of frozen water to roll down lower back
- Aromatherapy oils
- Small amount of plain massage oil
- Rebozo
- Fill a plastic water bottle two-thirds full, lay it on its side and freeze. In labour remove it from the freezer and add cold water. This will stay an icy drink for hours in the hospital.
- Ice cubes made from frozen juice
- Birth ball
- Rescue Remedy
- Plastic spray bottle of water to spritz face
- 2 flannels – one cold for face, one hot for perineum. Colour code them!
- LED candles
- Music
- Hypnobirth CD
- Her own pillow and blanket
- Lip balm
- Hair band
- Massage ball or tennis ball
- Small food – bite size
- Bikini top/tankini for wearing in the pool
- Kneeling pads for the pool

Birth Plans

What is a birth plan for?

A birth plan is a written plan of how you would like to give birth. Although it is impossible to know in advance what kind of experience you will have, it can be a good idea to think about some of the options you may face.

Writing a birth plan may help you to make informed choices about the care you receive, and will help to communicate your wishes with your birth partners and midwife.

A birth plan is not a contract to which you will be held if you change your mind, or your circumstances change. Try to be flexible about your birth plan, you can change or add to it as you wish.

What should be included in your birth plan?

You should include anything that is important to you for your birth experience. Things to consider including in your plan may be:

- Where you intend to give birth (home, midwife led unit or hospital)
- Who you want to be present at the birth (partner, friend, relatives)
- Whether you would like a student midwife to be involved in your care
- What techniques you want to use, if any (relaxation, hypnobirth, birth pool, aromatherapy, medicinal analgesia)
- Active birth
- Who is to cut the baby's umbilical cord
- Who is to check the sex of the baby first if you don't know
- How you want to give birth to the placenta (natural or managed)
- How you will feed your baby

- If you want your baby to have vitamin K
- Any special personal, spiritual or religious needs you may have

Who should see the birth plan?

It may help to write the birth plan with someone – usually your support person in labour. You can discuss your birth plan with any of your care providers at any stage in your pregnancy or labour, as they may be able to help you with some of your choices.

There is a space provided for your birth plan in your handheld notes, or you can write it separately and keep it with your notes. Once in labour ensure that your midwife reads the plan as she/he needs to know your birth preferences.

The 'Golden Hour'

Whenever possible it is important for your baby to have skin to skin contact, this is often referred to as the 'Golden Hour'. A huge amount of research has been done on the benefits of skin to skin contact. More than a decade ago Michel Odent wrote an article published in Midwifery Today, (2002) called "The First Hour Following Birth: Don't Wake the Mother!" In the article Odent describes twelve separate perspectives including:

- The sudden need to breathe
- The effects of hormones on bonding
- Helping to regulate the baby's temperature
- The bacteriological point of view
- The beginning of lactation

Babies will initiate feeding when they are ready and babies that are in skin to skin contact with their mother will normally breastfeed within the first hour. Contact with the chest area stimulates the brain through the sight of the nipple/areola developing neural pathways; as well as stimulating the olfactory senses which encourages both milk production and the urge to feed. As little as 20 minutes skin to skin has been shown to increase exclusive breastfeeding by 1.35 months and to delay weaning by 2.10 months. (Mikiel-Kostyra K, Mazur J, Bołtruszko I, 2002).

Nils Bergen is a physician from South Africa with a special interest in perinatal neuroscience and an advocate of skin to skin contact for all babies. He believes it is important so that mothers and their babies "can begin breastfeeding and bonding naturally, and to go on to establish a secure attachment relationship for a better society" – (http://www.skintoskincontact.com). Bergen suggests that as much as 1000 minutes (or 17 hours) skin to skin is needed in order for all the long-term benefits to be realised. Whilst this may not be practical in our modern lives, it is certainly thought provoking...

Another good resource on the benefits of skin to skin is: http://www.unicef.org.uk/BabyFriendly/Health-Professionals/Care-Pathways/Breastfeeding/Birth/

Whilst this skin to skin time is important, and if you can have it, then you should do everything you can to spend this time quietly, with soft lighting and gentle voices. Most hospitals actively encourage this and your midwife should support you to have this time. If you need medical attention this is the perfect time for birth partners to take over skin to skin which will encourage bonding for them too.

If however your baby needs to have medical attention which means that this contact is not possible, don't despair. Breastfeeding and bonding can be established later on although it may require more effort on your part. I'd like to share my own story with you, which in no small part led me to hypnotherapy and ultimately hypnobirth.

My son was born in 1986, when natural birth was considered to be rather "hippie-ish" and definitely not for the first time mother, I was very keen to have a birth without drugs. Unfortunately I became ill during my pregnancy and spent three months in hospital. The illness was not caused by the pregnancy, but towards the end I also developed pre-eclampsia. Shortly before my due date my blood pressure shot up and the decision was made to induce my baby. I was put on a drip overnight and the following morning the doctor broke my waters and they discovered that I had had a partial-abruption of the placenta. My surges began immediately and because of the drip they were very intense.

My son was born three and half hours later and he was having difficulty breathing. After a quick glimpse of him he was whisked away to the Special Care Unit and I didn't see him again for nearly 48 hours. We both gradually improved and after 10 days in hospital we were sent home. Although he was bottle fed for those first few days, I was determined to breastfeed and after a tricky start we got the hang of it.

Although we had recovered from the birth, my illness continued and when he was ten weeks old I went back into hospital for an operation.

In those days it wasn't seen as a priority to keep mother and baby together, so it was a week of being bottle fed before I saw him again. By this time he had changed so much that I didn't recognise him and accused my husband of bringing the wrong baby. A difficult moment!

Eventually I went home and although I began to recover physically I developed post-natal depression. I can honestly say that that first year was really tough, but thanks to some really great healthcare professionals I got through it and began to feel more like myself again. But it left me with a poor bond with my baby. When I picked him up he would often cry until I put him down again. I realise now that he was probably picking up on how bad I was feeling and it made him feel bad too.

One afternoon a few weeks after his first birthday I was talking to a very good friend and complained that I was sad that I didn't have a very cuddly baby – her baby loved to be cuddled. There was quite a long pause, and then she took a deep breath and told me sternly that as I was the adult in this relationship I should make the first move. I felt as if I had been given a real telling off, for which I will be eternally grateful. From that moment on I made a real effort every day to change the relationship I had with my baby in order to develop the bond. It was hard to begin with, but after a while I started to notice a difference and then our bond began to really grow and our relationship flourished. The relationship I have with my gorgeous son now couldn't be better.

The point of telling you this is that no matter what happens to get in the way of your ability to bond with your baby, it is possible. If you need it, get all the help you can from family, friends and professionals. And of course, if all goes well please make the most of those first precious hours to bond; to develop breastfeeding and to allow those neural pathways to form.

If you find your birth experience has been difficult please make an appointment for a debrief with your hospital maternity department. There will be specialist midwives who can take you through your notes and answer any questions you may have. For some women a seemingly straightforward experience can leave them with unresolved feelings. An unexpected caesarean birth can result in feelings of loss for the birth that was planned.

Skin to skin postnatally can be wonderful for both mum and baby. There is a technique which is growing in popularity called 'rebirthing'. This involves recreating the birth environment that you had planned. It can be done some time after birth, days or perhaps weeks.

Water allows a baby to reconnect with the womb environment. There may be a birth pool at home which was not used, or a bath. The room should be warm, the lights low, soft music, warm towels. Ideally the woman and baby should be supported by someone else, often the birth partner and/or a close friend.

The woman can be in the bath, and once comfortable the baby passed to her. The water should be body temperature (37 degrees). Allow the baby to be submerged up to the shoulders and to float, supporting his head. It can take about a minute for the baby to calm. Keep the lights low. Talk to baby. Consider playing the hypnobirth CD or music from your birth playlist. The baby can gently be moved to a skin to skin position with mum and will often breastfeed on demand. This is also a great way to overcome breastfeeding challenges.

The process of reconnecting with baby in this way, rebirthing, can result in emotion, sometimes tears. It is important to have a support person who understands why this is important and an opportunity to talk with someone after your birth.

Section SEVEN

Class Handouts and Home Practice

Class One

Affirmations

The Language of Hypnobirth

Positive Sign

Vicious Cycle

Your Breathing

Induction – Progressive Relaxation

Home Practice Week One

Affirmations

- With every out breath I can double my relaxation
- As I focus on my breathing my body responds with complete relaxation
- Each day I grow more and more confident that my birth will be calm and comfortable
- Every time I practice my relaxation it will be easier, quicker and deeper
- I feel my body softening, relaxing and releasing with every surge
- I trust my body and surrender to the process of birth
- I am a powerful woman
- My long slow out breath centres and calms me
- I welcome each surge and allow my body to open easily
- I allow myself to drift down and down, deeper and deeper
- My mind is focussed on a calm relaxed birth; I trust my body to follow
- My body and my baby are working instinctively together for a calm relaxed birth

Contd....

- Each surge takes me closer and closer to holding my baby
- I feel empowered, supported and confident to experience the birth that is right for me
- I trust my body to respond in a relaxed manner, no matter what direction my birth takes
- Release, relax, just let go
- Relax, relax, relax

The Language of Hypnobirth

Our words and thoughts shape our experience

Thoughts are the means by which we shape our experiences. We know that the mind reacts to language with emotion. The hypnobirth philosophy aims to use language that describes what is happening during the birthing experience in a gentler, non-medical manner.

We want to use words that evoke an emotion of feeling good, rather than fear and lack of understanding. Our words reinforce the belief that birth is a natural, normal life event.

Medicalised Language	**Hypnobirth Language**
Contraction	Surge
Pain	Sensation
Delivery	Birth
Pushing	Birth breathing
Effacing/Dilating	Thinning / Opening
Patients	Clients
Braxton Hicks	Pre-labour warm-ups
Fully dilated	Fully open
Sweep	Cervical massage
Primips / Multips	1st / 2nd time Mums
Transition	Near completion

Feel free to share your positive birth story.

If you have nothing nice to say, please say nothing at all!

Vicious Cycle of Stress, Tension and Pain in Labour

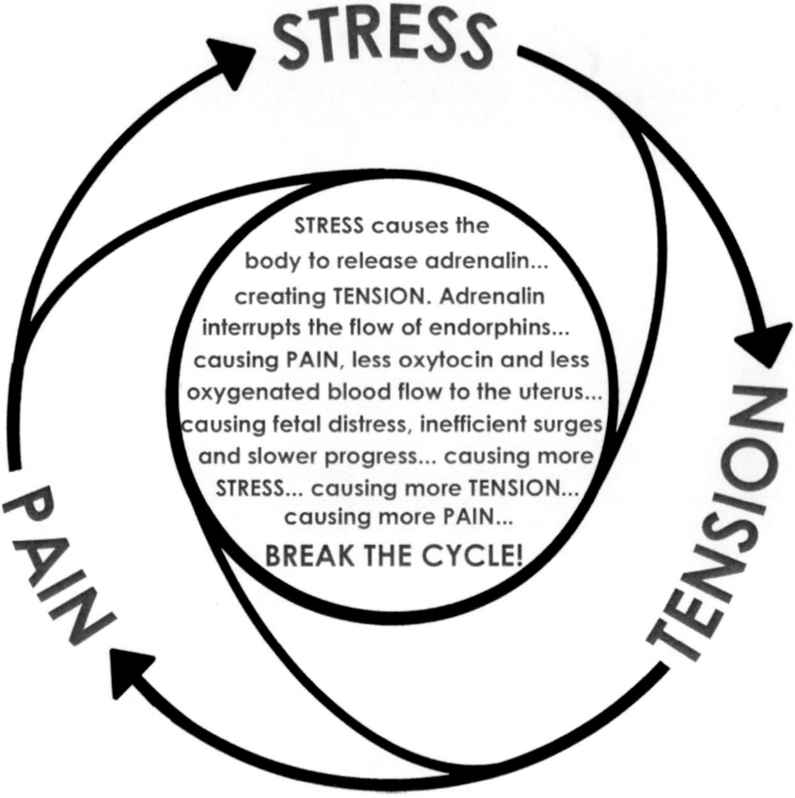

Your Breathing

Surge breathing for First Stage

Take a slow breath in through your nose. Breathe out through a soft loose mouth, making your out breath longer and slower than the in breath.

Relax your body with each out breath. Think about dropping your shoulders, relaxing your hands and keep your mouth and jaw tension free.

You may want to add counting to the breath. As you breathe in ask your birth partner to count. As you breathe out, focus on a longer count.

For example you may count to 3 as you breathe in, and 5 as you breathe out.

The length of your breath will increase as you practice. Use this breath in the first stage of labour during every surge to enable you to remain relaxed and calm.

You may like to imagine a big balloon in your belly. Give the balloon a colour if it helps. As you breathe in, the balloon inflates. As you breathe out the balloon deflates. See the balloon grow with each in breath.

The breath will allow your abdominal muscles to relax; this creates space as your uterus moves with each surge. The deep breathing increases oxygen and blood flow to the uterus, and therefore your baby. Muscles and diaphragm relax, and surges become more comfortable.

Practice this breathing for a few minutes twice a day.

J breathing for Second Stage

This breath encourages you to release and relax the pelvic floor area. Breath holding tightens and tenses the pelvic floor, holding your baby in.

Take a big quick breath in through your nose and, as you slowly release it through your nose, focus your breath downward towards your pelvic floor.

Visualise the 'J' shape.

You will know when your body wants to breathe the baby down. Helpful visualisations are the crowning rose.

This is not a practice breath, but can be used in the last 6 weeks of pregnancy on the loo.

Progressive Relaxation

Make yourself comfortable. Take a couple of nice deep breaths and when you're ready you can allow your eyes to gently close.

As you breathe in deeply and exhale slowly you can allow yourself to relax. Breathing in deeply, exhaling slowly and as you breath out you can allow your body to release, relax, just let go.

And as you begin to relax, you may become more aware of things around you, the sounds in the room, the sounds outside the room. Just allow all of these sounds to take you further and further into relaxation.

You may also become more aware of your thoughts, things that you need to do, but just take these few minutes for yourself now, and allow your thoughts to drift in and out of your mind easily. And if any thoughts keep coming back into your mind, put them in a bubble and allow them to float away, just for now... As you listen to the sound of my voice and allow yourself to drift further and further into relaxation, you can allow yourself to focus on what's important, peace, calm and relaxation.

Turning your attention to your head for a moment, allow a feeling of relaxation to develop in your head and face. Imagine the muscles of your scalp relaxing just by wanting it to happen it can happen.

Allow that feeling of relaxation to flow into your facial muscles now, relaxing your forehead, your eyebrows, the tiny muscles around your eyes. Relaxing your cheeks. Relaxing your ears.

Relaxing your mouth, and your jaw, relaxing your tongue.

You can allow this feeling of relaxation to flow down your neck, relaxing your neck and your throat, flowing into your shoulders now, releasing, relaxing, just let go.... You can allow a lovely, warm feeling to flow with this feeling of relaxation, softening and relaxing all of your muscles.

You can be interested to know whether this feeling of relaxation will move quickly or s l o w l y down your arms now, all the way down now, all the way down, right the way down to very tips of your fingers. Soft, warm, gentle relaxation. Release, relax, just let go.

Allow that feeling to flow down your back, releasing, relaxing the muscles on either side of your spine. Relaxing your chest, and allowing that feeling to flow down into your torso now. Relaxing your stomach, the muscles of your pelvic area, just as you will when you give birth to our baby. Release, relax, just let go.

Now, allowing that feeling to flow through your pelvis and your hips into your legs. Relaxing your legs, your thighs, your calves and your shins. You can allow a feeling of heaviness to develop in your legs and the heavier they become the more relaxed you can feel. The more relaxed you feel the heavier they can become, allowing you to sink further and further into relaxation.

Now you can stay in this feeling of relaxation as long as you want. Resting in this space where time means nothing – an hour seems like a minute. A minute is just a blink. Rest in this space, relax, relax, relax.

Contd...

[If it's bedtime, read this paragraph] Now allow yourself to drift into a beautiful peaceful night's sleep.

[Otherwise, read this paragraph] In a moment it will be time to come back into the room, feeling confident and relaxed, knowing that each time you do this you will find it easier and easier to relax and you will feel more and more confident about the birth of our/your baby. So you can begin by moving your fingers and toes and very gently, in your own time you can gently open your eyes, feeling great.

Home Practice – Week One

Daily breathing practice. Close your eyes- breathe into your abdomen as you inhale and release your breath twice as slowly. Use the balloon visualisation if that helps. Practice as often as you can over the next week, getting used to the sensation of diaphragmatic breathing!

Start listening to your relaxation CD. Try before bed to help you sleep. Begin with a few long slow breaths then allow yourself to drift with the relaxation.

Begin to avoid watching programmes or films portraying birth badly. These programs are ***not*** harmless entertainment. We will watch positive hypnobirths in class.

From now on, avoid conversations on birth which you know are going to end badly. You know who those people are! If someone wishes to share a positive birth story then great. If not they can keep it until after you have given birth.

List any questions, thoughts or worries you have. Bring the list to the next session.

Cut up your affirmations and put them where you visit several times a day. This could be the inside of kitchen cupboards where you keep the cups, or where you brush your teeth. When you see them, repeat them aloud (or whisper to yourself!) to really anchor them in.

If you cannot connect with them, write your own!

Class Two

Raspberry Leaf Tea

The Third Stage of Labour

Perineal Massage

Changing the Threshold of Labour Sensation

Fear Release Exercise (Pt. 1)

Staircase Deepener

Home Practice Week Two

Raspberry Leaf Tea

Raspberry leaf tea is a herbal remedy that has been in traditional use for many years. It will not be suitable for everyone, and although we view it as herbal it contains powerful natural chemicals. It should not be confused with fruit tea.

The raspberry plant (*Rubus idaeus*) belongs to the rose family. Red raspberry leaves contain the phytochemical fragarine, which is the active constituent responsible for toning the muscles of the uterus. The leaves also contain organic iron, which is easily absorbed by the body, helping to prevent anaemia (Campion, 1996). The astringency of the leaves is due to the tannin content, which helps prevent haemorrhage, as well as toning and strengthening the tissues of the reproductive organs and preventing bleeding gums, a common feature of pregnancy.

The raspberry works on the smooth muscle of the uterus to give it ***tone.*** It increases the strength of the myometrium, facilitating an easier birth. **It is not a tea to induce labour.** It is meant to make the surges more efficient. If you are considering taking raspberry leaf tea buy the loose tea or teabags rather than the tablets. The taste is not to everyone's liking!

You should always tell your midwife you are taking raspberry leaf tea.

Precautions – Do **not** *take raspberry leaf tea if:*

- You are anaemic and are taking iron supplements
- You are having more than one baby
- Your baby is in the breech position
- You are planning a caesarean birth or have experienced a previous caesarean birth
- You have experienced bleeding in pregnancy
- You have experienced a very rapid birth (less than 3 hours) previously

- You have experienced premature birth before
- If you are taking antidepressants
- If you have high blood pressure
- If you have any medical complications

How to take the tea

Raspberry leaf has an accumulative effect. This means ideally begin at around 32 weeks' gestation. Start with one cup a day. It may be that you experience some Braxton Hicks. If they become strong, reduce your intake. You can gradually build to 3 cups a day.

During early or pre labour you can sip hot tea at home. Some women like to make ice cubes with it to suck in labour.

The Royal College of Midwives respects the rights and choices of women to either self-administer complementary and alternative medicines or to seek the advice, counsel and treatment from complementary and alternative practitioners.

The Third Stage of Labour

The third stage of labour is the time from the birth of the baby to the expulsion of the placenta and membranes

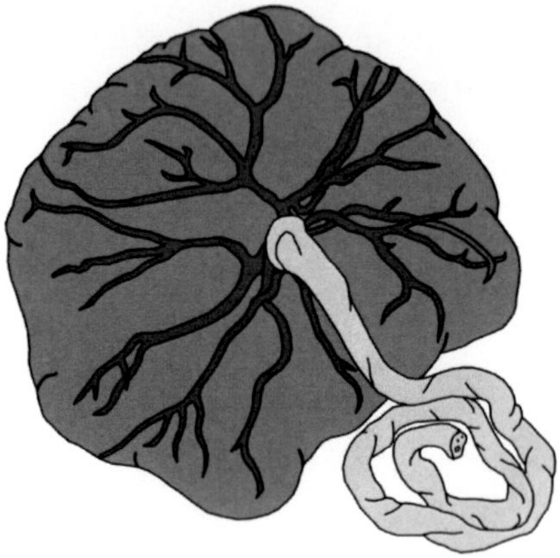

In the womb the baby's blood circulates from baby to the placenta through 2 umbilical arteries and back through 1 umbilical vein. At full term at any one time one third to half of the baby's blood volume is in the placenta and cord.

In the first seconds after birth between 54-160mls of warm oxygenated blood that may have been held back by compression of the blood vessels during the birth flows from the placenta to the baby.

As the uterus contracts down more blood is pushed from the placenta to the baby. Some of this blood then returns to the placenta and a to-and-fro process takes places with the blood moving between baby and placenta. Eventually the blood exchange ensures that the newborn blood volume is equilibrated. This takes around 2-4 minutes but can be longer. The baby is essentially regulating his or her blood volume.

An unclamped cord helps the placenta to empty. It therefore loses blood volume, becomes smaller and detaches from the uterus more easily. It is easier to birth.

Even a small delay in clamping of the cord will be beneficial. The placental transfusion happens very quickly in the first minute after birth.

- Baby receives up to 50% extra blood volume
- Stem cell benefits
- Iron benefits – 30g of increased iron

NICE states that women who request a natural third stage and are low risk of haemorrhage should be supported in their decision.

Managed	***Natural***
NICE recommends clamping the cord between 1 and 5 minutes for a managed third stage	A true natural third stage can take place only if the cord is not clamped until after the mother has birthed her baby's placenta
A managed third stage:	**A natural third stage:**
Can shorten the third stage compared with a natural third stage	Can take longer (but not always)
Is associated with nausea and vomiting in about 100 in 1000 women	Is associated with nausea and vomiting in about 50 in 1000 women
Is associated with an approximate risk of 13 in 1000 of a haemorrhage of more than 1litre	Is associated with an approximate risk of 29 in 1000 of a haemorrhage of more than 1litre
Is associated with an approximate risk of 14 in 1000 of a blood transfusion	Is associated with an approximate risk of 40 in 1000 of a blood transfusion
Oxytocic drugs are administered with the woman's consent. The cord is clamped and cut. Once the midwife knows the placenta is ready to be birthed she uses controlled cord traction	No oxytocic drugs are used. The cord is left unclamped. The woman produces her own oxytocin which signals the placenta is ready. The woman births the placenta by pushing it out. The cord is then clamped and cut

NICE (2014)

Perineal Massage

A large study looked at the research that has been undertaken in perineal massage and found that massaging your perineum (the area between the vagina and the anus) in the antenatal period and during at least the last four weeks of pregnancy before your baby's due date, reduces the likelihood of tearing, and in particular, the need to be cut (episiotomy). This is because the better you prepare the muscle and tissues of the perineum for stretching; the less likely it is that the skin will tear.

- Wash your hands thoroughly
- Sit in a private, warm and comfortable place
- Apply a lubricant such as KY jelly, olive oil or unscented massage oil to your hands and the perineal area
- Place both thumbs around 3cm/1½ inches (around half the length of your thumb) into the vagina. You could start gently by using one thumb
- Massage the area by gently rubbing the perineal tissues between your thumbs and fingers
- Press downwards and to the sides, gently stretching until you feel a tingling or slightly 'burning' sensation, this feeling lessens after a few moments. Discontinue if you experience pain
- Once this sensation is felt, hold the stretch for around one minute until the feeling subsides and begin gently massaging the lower part of the vagina by moving your thumbs back and forth. While massaging also hook your thumbs onto the sides of the vagina and gently pull these tissues forward, as the baby's head does when it is being born

- Continue to gently rub as you stretch for around three to four minutes

By massaging the perineum like this once a day, you will notice the area becoming more flexible and you will become more accustomed to the stretching sensations which occur during birth.

What Else Helps?

Perineal massage alone is not the only technique that can help women have a labour without an episiotomy or serious tear, other preventative measures include:

- Pelvic floor exercises - a muscle that is used is better prepared to stretch than one which is tight and unrelenting

- Squatting which works with gravity, increases pelvic diameter by 10%, shortens the depth of the birth canal, shortens second stage of labour and decreases the need for instrumental delivery and episiotomy. These benefits are achieved because squatting tilts the uterus and pelvis forward placing the baby in the proper alignment for birth. Squatting encourages and strengthens the intensity of contractions whilst relieving back pressure and helps relax and stretch the pelvic floor muscles

- Home birth. A study by Murphy and Feinland in New York of 1068 women who had home births 69.6% had intact perineums

- Slow controlled birth is another key to an intact perineum and reduced incidence of laceration. The birthing woman must listen to her body, working with her breath to birth the baby. Breath holding and pushing work against the body and increase the likelihood of tearing

Changing the Threshold of Labour Sensation

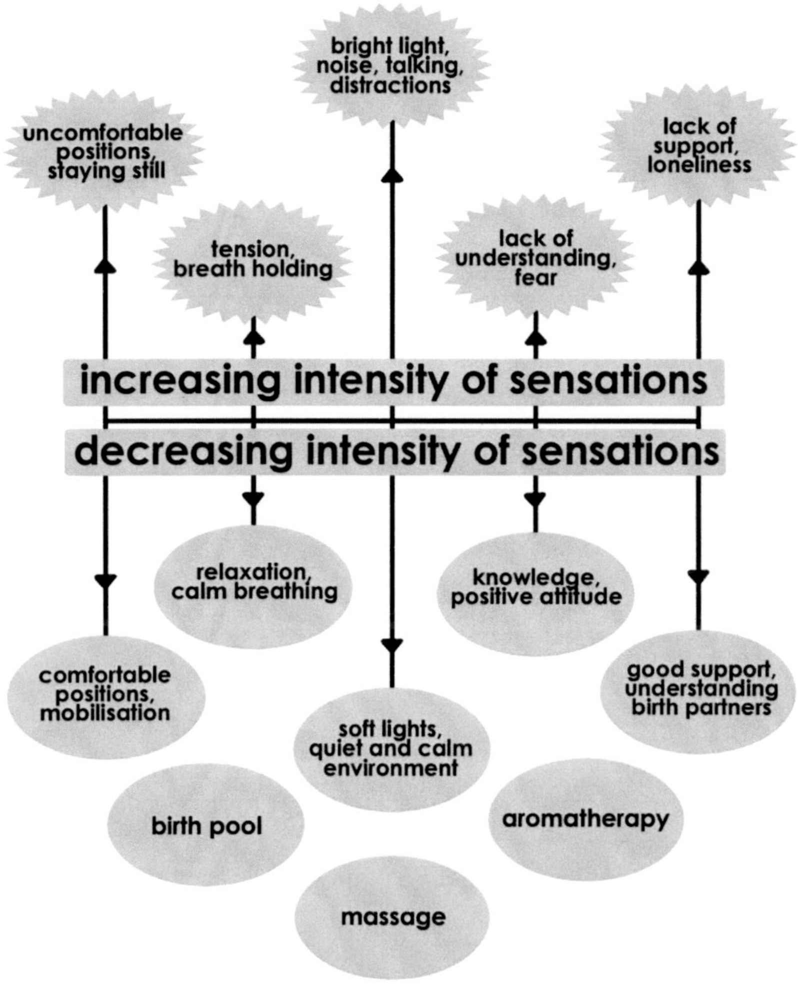

Anxiety Release Exercise

Sit quietly and consider any fears/anxieties or limiting thoughts you have around birth. Write them below, and score them on a scale of 1 - 5

1 – A bit anxious
5 – Very anxious

The birth partner should do the same. Once completed, compare and discuss. We will use a fear release script in the next class.

Concerns / Issues / Anxieties / Thoughts	**Rating** **1 – 5**

Concerns / Issues / Anxieties / Thoughts	Rating 1 – 5

Staircase Deepener

In a moment I'm going to begin relaxing you further. In a moment I'm going to begin counting backwards from 10 to 1.

When I say the number 10, you can imagine in your mind's eye that you are standing at the top of a flight of 10 stairs.

As I say each number you will simply move down those stairs, relaxing more and more completely. At the bottom of the stairs is a path which you can walk along easily, calmly and comfortably. Even though you can't see exactly what's ahead of you along the path or around the corner you can be confident in your own ability and stay relaxed, calm and comfortable.

When I say the number 1 you will step onto the path and take the first step of your journey.

In labour, if you notice anyone touch you or move you this will allow you to relax even more. Deeper and deeper, more and more relaxed.

So, breathe in deeply, and we can begin

10, at the top of the stairs, you're relaxing and letting go, 10

9, becoming more relaxed, release, relax just let go, 9

8, sinking into a more comfortable, peaceful and relaxed position

You may notice sounds around you, simply allow these sounds to take you further and further into relaxation. Deeper and deeper, more and more relaxed

10

Contd....

9

8, 7 way down now

7

6

5 that's fine, you're doing perfectly, deeper and deeper

4

3

2 Deeper and deeper, more and more relaxed

5 down and down

4

3

2 way down now

3

2 way down now

3

2

On the next number 1 simply sink into a more comfortable, calm, peaceful and relaxed position

3

2

and 1... way down

Contd....

That's fine, you're doing perfectly. Now walk along the path and take yourself to a beautiful place in nature and relax. Provide yourself with everything you need to relax – a big squashy sofa, a hammock or even a feather bed. Make the temperature just right for you. Relax in this place and know that every time you come back here you can relax more deeply and more easily than before. Just by focussing on this place and taking a couple of deep breaths you can be transported into this feeling of relaxation.

In labour, if you notice any sounds around you or if anyone moves or touches you, this will allow you to relax even more. Deeper and deeper, more and more relaxed.

Now you can stay in this feeling of relaxation as long as you want. Resting in this space where time means nothing – an hour seems like a minute. A minute is just a blink. Rest in this space, relax, relax, relax.

[If it's bedtime, read this paragraph] Now allow yourself to drift into a beautiful peaceful night's sleep.

[Otherwise, read this paragraph] In a moment it will be time to come back into the room, feeling confident and relaxed, knowing that each time you do this you will find it easier and easier to relax and you will feel more and more confident about the birth of our/your baby. So you can begin by moving your fingers and toes and very gently, in your own time you can gently open your eyes, feeling great.

Home Practice – Week Two

Practice your breathing – Find some time each day. On the train, perhaps? Three breaths when waking? A good tip is to practice breathing during adverts on TV, or whilst sitting at a red traffic light!

Perineal massage practice – you can do this from about 32 weeks of pregnancy. Start looking for some unscented massage oil. www.elastolabo.co.uk

Pelvic floor exercises – it is good practice to start these soon. Try beginning with sets of 10. Find a trigger. Every time you go upstairs, sitting at traffic lights, waiting for your laptop to fire up

Raspberry leaf tea – to tone the uterus. If you are considering this then 32 weeks is the ideal time to begin. Read the guidance on usage

Complete the Fear Release Exercise at home ready for next week's script

Consider buying a birth ball. We will practice positions next week

Class Three

Active Birth

Aromatherapy Oils for Labour

Massage for Birth

Shoulder Anchor

Induction of Labour

Top Tips for Spontaneous Labour

Home Practice Week Three

Active Birth

When the pelvis is upright it gains 28% more space!!

Standing leaning against the wall

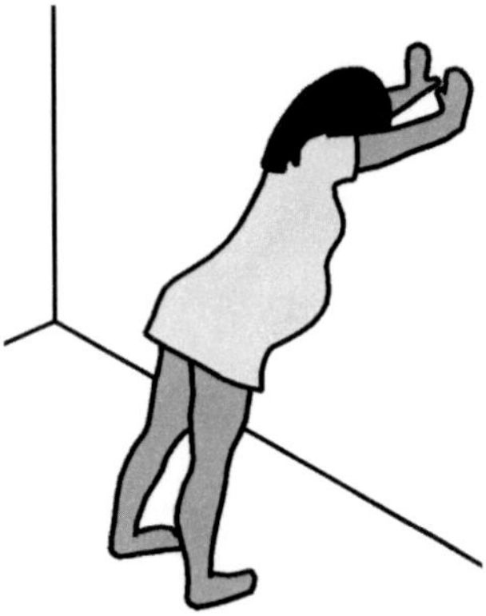

With the birth partner standing behind, and with the flat of the hand use long strokes from nape of neck to sacrum. Maintain contact at all times

Sacral pressure – heel of hand over sacrum. Woman leans into it, apply counter pressure

Standing Rebozo position

Birth partner moves with her breath

Add a ball behind her and lean against the wall

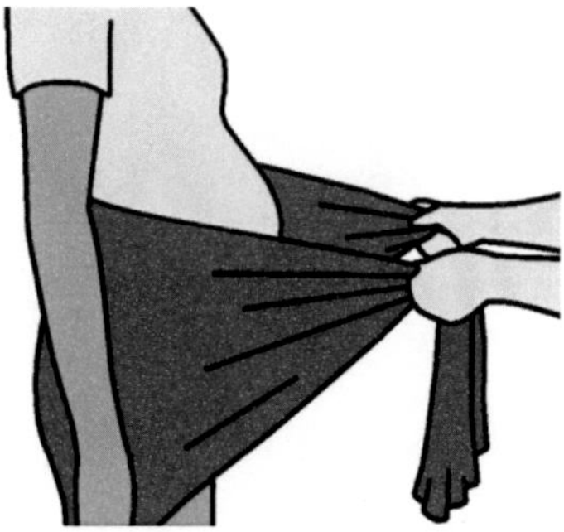

Using Your Birth Ball

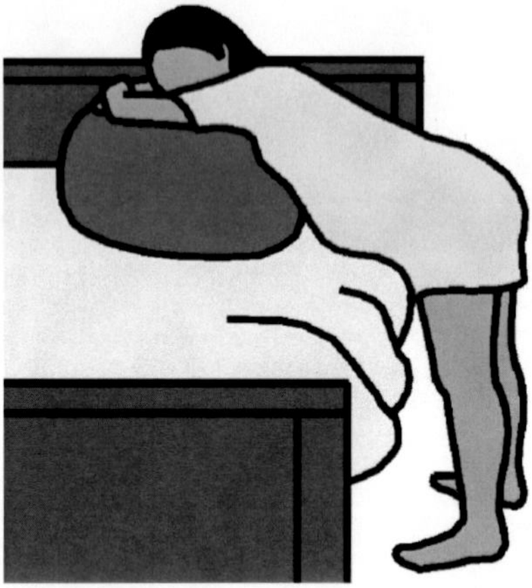

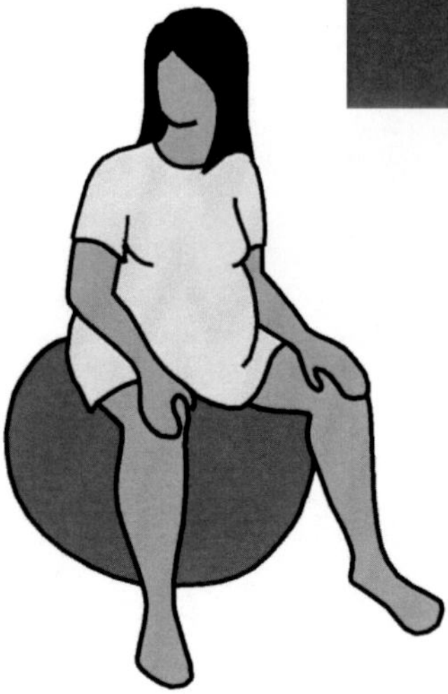

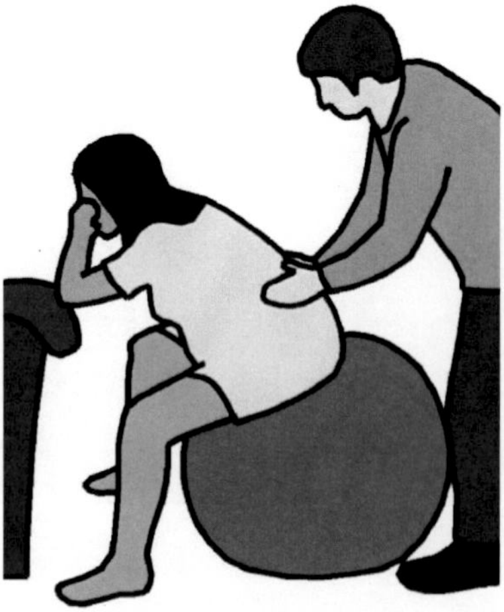

Hanging / Sitting Rebozo

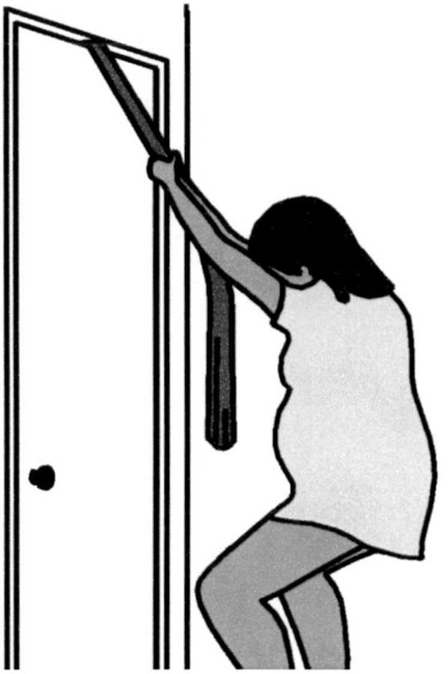

Hanging Rebozo to assist gravity

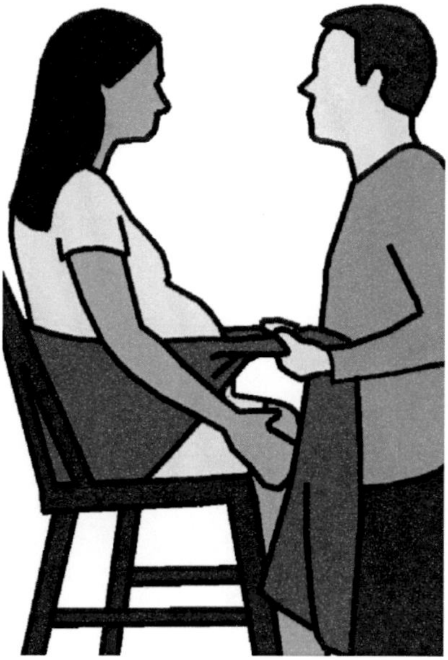

Sitting Rebozo to encourage relaxation

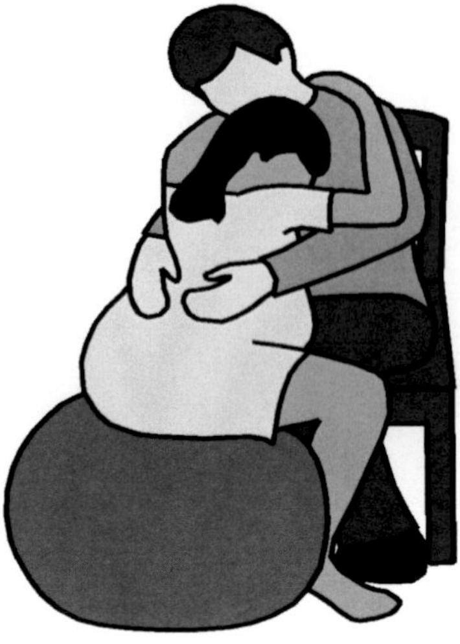

Forward leaning positions allow access to the back

Introduce light touch massage and the breath / shoulder anchor

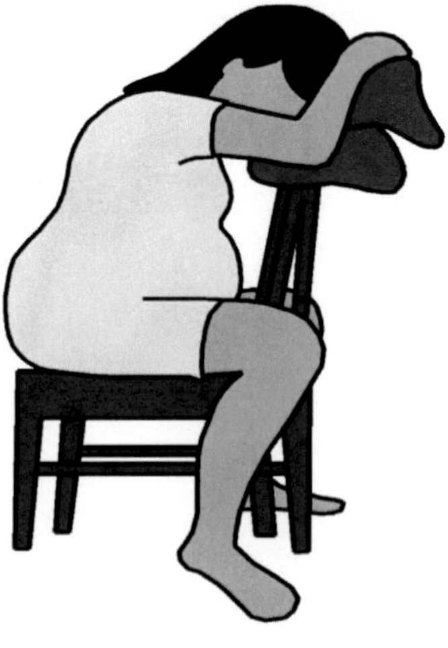

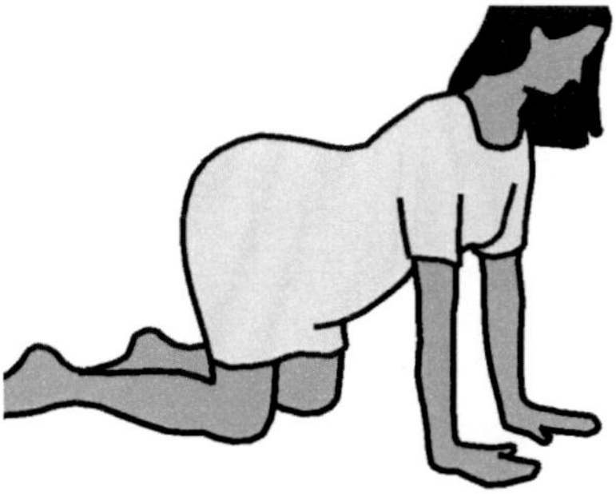

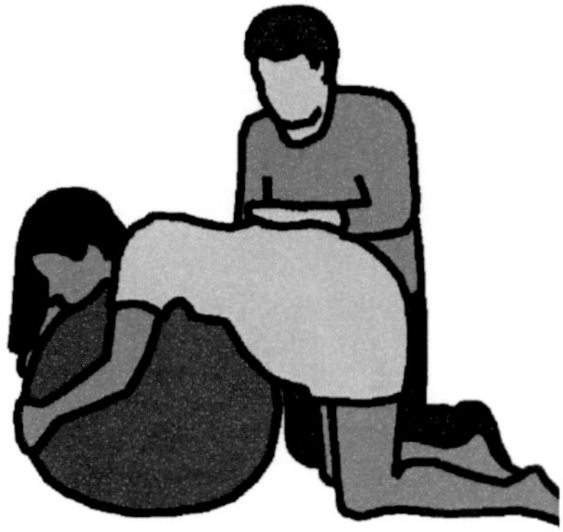

Introduce Sacral Massage

Shaking the Apples

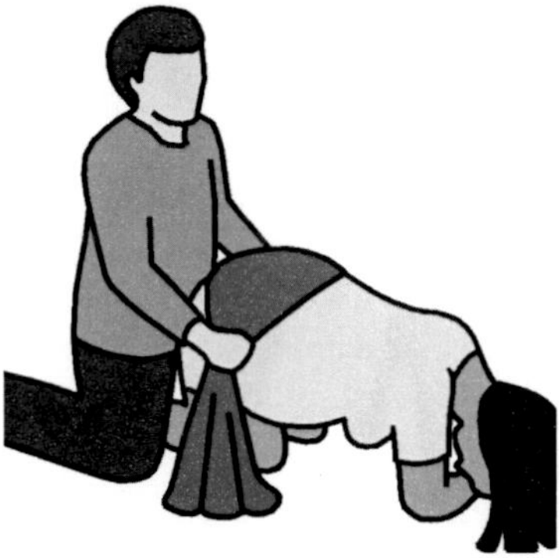

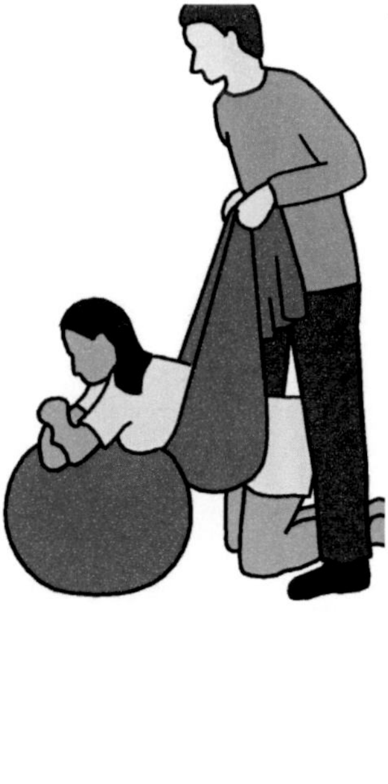

Sifting

Aromatherapy oils for labour

Dosage: 1 drop of oil to each 5ml of carrier oil

Bergamot – A*nalgesia, relieves fear, uplifting*

Jasmine – *Can help to dull the pressure and strengthen surges, thus shortening labour. Calming, energising and uplifting*
reduces stress, enhances uterine action, acceleration of labour
Can be overpowering. Consider effect on birth partner and midwife.
Buy purest oil possible

Lavender – *Relaxing and calming*
reduces anxiety, tension, enhances uterine action
Avoid with hay fever/asthma triggered by flower pollen. Not to be used with epidural anaesthetic due to potential interaction with bupivacaine.
Caution with induction of labour due to possible effect on uterine tone.
Be aware of sedative effect on partner and midwife

Neroli – *Reduces fear, apprehension and anxiety*
gently uplifting, relieves nausea, reduces anxiety

Rose – *A fab tonic for the system, helps deepen and calm breathing and assists the circulation*
analgesia, calming, reduces fear
Late pregnancy only. Great mixed with lavender

Frankincense – *Good for transition of labour*
Calming. Balances emotion, releases fear. Avoid if asthmatic

Clary sage – *Great tension reliever. Euphoric and heady – use in moderation, but great during birthing*

To be used ONLY if after 40 weeks

1 drop on a tissue and inhale

For lower back ache in labour

Add 1-4 drops (+ 1 drop Clary Sage and 1 drop Jasmine or lavender) to 300ml of warm water, immerse a cloth / flannel compress and apply to lower back

If using oils in the bath, put into full-fat milk first to disperse the oil

Maximum 6 drops added to either 15mls carrier oil or 15mls full fat milk (recommended)

Not in birth pools

For vaporisation 2-4 drops of oil in a bowl of warm water

Massage for Labour

Stroking back massage – whole hand flat at nape of neck. Move hand firmly down to sacrum. Use other hand to begin again, ensuring you never break contact.

- Good for in between surges

Sacral pressure. Find the sacrum with the heel of your hand. Support the sacrum. Encourage your partner to push back onto your hand as firmly as she feels comfortable. Let HER dictate the pressure.

- Good for during a surge

Light touch massage 1

Begin at the sacrum. Use the backs of your fingers, beginning in the middle and working out to form a 'V' shape. Work your way up her back, always include the nape of her neck. Once at her neck begin working down in the same 'V' shape. DO NOT take your hands from the top to start again at the sacrum.

- Good with a surge

Light touch massage 2

Begin at the sacrum. Use the tips of your fingers. Imagine a side lying '8'. Cross the 8 at the spine. Allow your fingers to elongate the 8, and take it all the way out to her sides. Work your way up the back, into the nape of the neck. Work back down.

- Good for more intense/quicker surges

Breath Anchoring

- As she breathes **IN**, run the tips/backs of your fingers up either side of her spine
- As she breathes **OUT,** place your hands firmly on each shoulder and anchor down for **all** of her out breath
- Repeat
- Allow your hands to follow her breath
- Breathe with her

Shoulder Anchor

I am going to begin with my hand in front of your eyes. As my hand moves I would like you to follow it ***only*** with your eyes. Keep your head still. *[**hold hand above her head**].*

Now focus your attention on my hand. Stare at it. As you do your eyes begin to feel very dry. Your eyes are becoming heavy. You feel as though you want to blink. Your eyes are heavy and tired, as though they want to close. Please resist the temptation to close your eyes.

I am going to slowly bring my hand down ***[begin to lower hand]*** and as it passes your face just allow your eyes to close and bring yourself into a wonderfully relaxed state.... Deeply relaxed..... Anytime I place my hand on your shoulder with a gentle downward pressure you will double your relaxation. *[**use shoulder anchor**]*

*[**remove hand**]* As you rest, allow your breathing to slow and deepen........

Now, become aware of your forehead....... Allow your forehead to smooth and relax.

Now, become aware of your eyes, gently closed. Feel all the little muscles in and around your eyes relaxing. This relaxation flows down and around your mouth, down into your jaw, which loosens and relaxes. With your next long slow out breath allow all tension in your body to release and relax.

Contd....

When you next feel my hand on your shoulder you will double your relaxation. ***[use shoulder anchor]*** Deeply relaxed. ***[remove hand]***

Now you will feel me lift your arm. ***[take hold of her thumb and lift arm above her lap]*** Allow me to take the weight of your arm, just let your arm go limp. In a moment I'm going to drop your arm onto your lap. When your arm drops down onto your leg you will double your relaxation. ***[drop arm onto her lap]***

Once again I am going to lift your arm. Just let your arm go limp. ***[lift arm].*** As I drop your arm this time you will bring yourself twice as deep into relaxation. Doubling your relaxation ***[drop arm]***

And once more I will lift your arm and drop it. ***[lift arm]*** and as you feel your arm drop you will experience deeper relaxation ..... Deeper than before. ***[drop arm]***

Anytime I place my hand on your shoulder ***[use shoulder anchor]*** with a gentle downward pressure you will double you relaxation. When you feel my hand on your shoulder next time you will feel calm, confident and relaxed. ***[remove hand].*** And now I will count from 1 up to 5....

1 ....beginning to become aware of your surroundings....

2 .... 3 ....eyelids feel lighter....

4 ....hands beginning to move....

5 ....eyes open return to the room feeling relaxed and confident.

Induction of Labour

Coming into hospital for induction of labour may not be the kind of experience you planned for. However there is much you can do to work with your body and baby.

- On arrival at hospital try to eliminate any stressors. If you are uncertain of a procedure/equipment/medical terminology just ask
- **Pull the curtains around the bed for privacy**
- Play some music. Earphones would be great
- Bring books/magazines to read
- **Bring nice food**
- Have some aromatherapy oils in a plastic spray bottle. Spritz your pillow for instant relaxation
- Massage techniques encourage relaxation. Light touch massage, a foot/hand/head massage would be wonderful

If you need to stay overnight:

- Feel free to display your pictures
- **Why not bring your own pillow from home?**
- Go out for a walk as often as you like
- Find the restaurant for dinner
- Order food in

Top Tips for Spontaneous Labour

Baby needs to be in a good position for labour to start – head down and low onto the cervix. By 37 weeks plan to use your ball to encourage baby down. Spend the evening sitting on the ball to watch TV. Try leaning over the ball with cushions under your knees and rock.

Pregnancy yoga, pilates and aquanatal will also help with the positioning of baby.

Relaxation will promote endorphins and oxytocin – your labour hormones. Practice your breathing techniques. Warm baths, massage and laughter all help with relaxation.

Cervical massage (sweep) can increase your chances of spontaneous labour. Discuss this with your midwife.

Try acupuncture

Try a date night. Go out for dinner. Kissing, laughing, foreplay all help.

Sex, sex and some more sex if you can manage it! Orgasms and nipple stimulation both produce large amounts of oxytocin.

Home Practice – Week Three

Birth partners – have you read a script yet? Practice with the progressive relaxation

Practice anchoring techniques – Shoulder anchor

Practice light touch massage

Use your birth ball for optimal baby positioning

Are your affirmations up? If not why not?!

Class Four

Breathing Scripts:

- Golden Thread
- Eye of the Storm
- Ice Cube

Eyes Opening & Closing

Birth Partner's Guide

Birth Partners Birthing Prompts

Room Sign

BRAIN – Informed Choice

Birth Plan Notes

Your Birth Plan

Hand Anaesthesia Anchor

Home Practice Week Four

Golden Thread

Make yourself comfortable and when you are ready, allow your eyes to gently close. Relax your face, especially your jaw.

Breathe in through your nose and gently out through your mouth, keeping your teeth and lips softly parted. Take a moment to establish this gentle way of breathing, making sure that the breath is flowing easily and comfortably. Notice the rhythm of your breathing.

Imagine a surge beginning. As it does, take a normal breath in through the nose, then breathe out very gently through the mouth. Feel a soft gentle breeze passing between your lips and imagine that on this soft breeze is fine golden thread flowing out between your lips.

Allow your mouth to open just enough to blow the thread away.

Keep your mind on this golden thread until the end of your out-breath, then allow the next in-breath to come of its own accord. Continue to breathe in this way, allowing the out-breath to lengthen quite naturally a little more each time.

With each out breath notice how you can blow the thread a little further away from you, using your breath to extend the thread further and further into the distance.

Breathing in deeply, filling your lungs with oxygen, exhaling slowly, your out breath is long and slow as the golden thread flows out in front of you. Watch in your mind, the beautiful thread drifting further and further away with each breath.

When you are ready, allow your breathing to return to normal and bring your awareness back to the room.

Eye of the Storm

Make yourself comfortable and allow your eyes to gently close. Relax your face, especially your jaw.

Breathe in through your nose and gently out through your mouth, keeping your teeth and lips softly parted. Take a moment to establish this gentle way of breathing, making sure that the breath is flowing easily and comfortably. Notice the rhythm of your breathing.

Imagine a surge beginning. As it does, take a normal breath in through the nose, then breathe out very gently through the mouth.

As you continue to breathe in and out through soft lips, imagine yourself at the centre of a storm where the air is still and everything remains calm. All around the storm rages, swirling wind and torrential rain. But here, in the eye of the storm, you are peaceful and calm.

No matter what goes on around you in the storm, here in the quiet, tranquil centre you remain calm and peaceful. Focus on your out breath then allow the next in-breath to come of its own accord. Continue to breathe in this way, allowing the out-breath to slow and lengthen quite naturally a little more each time. Continue breathing in and breathing out. Breathing in and breathing out.

You are aware of the power of the storm. You may hear noises from the wind around, but you remain centred in your own private space, quiet and calm, your long slow out breath relaxing and releasing the surge.

The surge begins to fade, and as it does you let the image of the storm fade, allowing your breathing to return to normal.

Ice Cube

Make yourself comfortable and allow your eyes to gently close. Relax your face, especially your jaw.

Breathe in through your nose and gently out through your mouth keeping your teeth and lips softly parted. Take a moment to establish this gentle way of breathing, making sure that the breath is flowing easily and comfortably. Notice the rhythm of your breathing.

Imagine a surge beginning. As it does, take a normal breath in through the nose, then breathe out very gently through the mouth.

Focus on the out breath, allow it to be longer and slower than your in breath. As you continue to focus on your out breath, imagine an ice cube in front of you.

Each time you breathe out, the warm air from your breath melts a little of the ice.

With each out breath watch the ice cube melt a little bit more, becoming smaller and smaller.

You can see a pool of melted water at its base, becoming larger and larger with each long slow out breath.

Keep focusing on your long slow out breath as the surge reaches its peak, then begins to fade.

Gradually the surge fades. The ice cube becomes smaller and smaller, and eventually both disappear and your breathing returns to normal.

In a moment it will be time to bring your awareness back to the room. You can begin to move your fingers and toes, and when you are ready you can gently open your eyes.

Eyes Opening and Closing

In a moment I'm going to count backwards from 99, I'd like you to count with me in your head. Closing your eyes on the odd the numbers and opening them on the even numbers.

So....

99 – Close your eyes and concentrate on your eyelids. Each and every time you close your eyes .... your eyelids will feel a little heavier

98 – Open your eyes ***[Then almost immediately count 97]***

97 – Close your eyes again and notice that your eyelids are beginning to feel that wonderful feeling of heaviness

96 – Open your eyes

95 – Close your eyes again, heavier and heavier, more and more relaxed ***[Leave the eyes closed for a little longer]***

94

93 – And closed. Becoming so relaxed and heavy that it's becoming more and more difficult to open them

92

91 – Closed. When you feel so relaxed that it's too much effort to bother to open your eyes you can allow them to stay closed, resting comfortably more and more relaxed

90

89 – Close your eyes again, heavier and heavier, more and more relaxed

Contd...

88

87 – And closed, going all the way down now , all the way down

86

85 – Closed, heavier and heavier, more and more relaxed. Really allowing that heaviness to flow through you now

84

83 – Closed, relax, relax, relax

82

81 – Closed letting it go now, letting it go, good...... Keeping your eyes closed now drifting further and further into relaxation

Now you can stay in this feeling of relaxation as long as you want. Resting in this space where time means nothing – an hour seems like a minute. A minute is just a blink. Rest in this space, relax, relax, relax.

Confident in the knowledge that you can return to this feeling of relaxation whenever you choose, by simply breathing, counting and just letting go.

[If it's bedtime, read this paragraph] Now allow yourself to drift into a beautiful peaceful night's sleep.

[Otherwise, read this paragraph] In a moment it will be time to come back into the room, feeling confident and relaxed, knowing that each time you do this you will find it easier and easier to relax and you will feel more and more confident about the birth of our/your baby. So you can begin by moving your fingers and toes and very gently, in your own time you can gently open your eyes, feeling great.

Birth Partner's Guide

When labour starts

During the night	Sleep until surges are 5-6 min apart
Position	Any position that's comfortable
Breathing	First stage surge breathing

During the day

Continue with normality. This might be a trip out, walks, eat and drink well. Early labour scripts. Baths, massage, aromatherapy, music. Build a nest

Start surge breathing early. Use balloon visualisation

Hypnobirth CD

Maybe go out for lunch/coffee?

Relax through surges – call midwife when surges are 5 minutes apart or when you need advice

Preparing home / hospital environment

Ask midwife to read the birth plan. Hypnobirth sign on the door

Dim the lights. Music, smells. Arrange room to promote Active Birth – birth ball/mat/birth stool/beanbag

Return home if less than 4 cm opened. Tune into body and baby

As Labour progresses

Keep mum well hydrated – offer small snacks for energy

Suggest frequent sitting on the toilet. A full bladder slows labour

Change position frequently to help rotate baby

Hydrotherapy – warm baths or showers help

Massage techniques to release endorphins

Rebozo

Surge breathing/3 step touch/counting and breathing techniques

Visualise filling a balloon

Second Stage

Mum expresses need to change breathing pattern

Mum assumes whatever position she is comfortable in for J-breathing

Mum follows the lead of her body, breathing down in a J-breath

No breath holding or 'pushing'. No prompts unless requested

Hot compress for perineum?

Shoulder anchor between surges?

Birth Partner's Birthing Prompts

These are the suggestions for the birth companion to use –softly and at random.

Between surges – useful phrases and *techniques*

- Long slow out breath. Relax with each breath out
- Every muscle limp and at ease; just relax your shoulders - release, relax, let go
- Relax and trust your body to know what to do
- Use counting and breathing techniques
- Use the shoulder anchor?
- Has she used the birth ball?

During Surges

- Body totally limp; go with your breathing
- Trust your body; long deep breaths
- Fill the balloon; give it a colour; fill it higher, higher
- SLOW breath up, fill the balloon up, up, up
- You may not have noticed how amazing your breathing was during that surge
- Release and relax downward now

During Second Stage J-Breathing

- Is she in a good position?
- Do what your body instinctively tells you
- Listen to your body
- Nudge your baby gently down to birthing
- Gently, softly breathe down to our baby
- Remind her to 'let go' and open

If not in water, consider a hot perineal compress

Room Sign

Hypnobirthing Room

- Please use low voices inside and outside our room — whisper if possible
- Please direct all conversation towards the birth partner unless absolutely necessary
- Please do not mention pain relief. If I need anything I will ask
- We would like the lights low
- We plan on using active birth and upright birth positions
- Allow me to use my natural birthing instincts to facilitate the movement of my baby
- I plan on using mother directed bearing down. Please — no valsalva breath holding

Thank you for your kind understanding and for sharing our day

BRAIN – Informed Choice

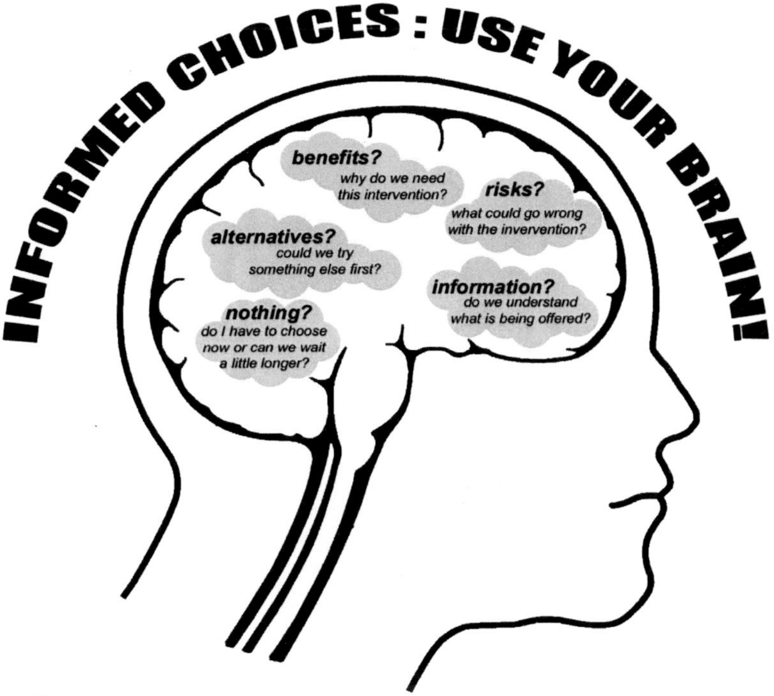

B = benefits — what are the benefits to mother and baby?

R = risks — what are the risks to mother and baby

A = alternatives — are there any alternative options?

I = information — do we have enough information to choose?

N = nothing — what happens if we do nothing or wait an hour?

Birth Plan Notes

What is a birth plan?

A birth plan is a written plan of how you would like to give birth. Although it is impossible to know in advance what kind of experience you will have, it can be a good idea to think about your choices.

Writing a birth plan may help you to think about the care you receive, and will help to share your wishes with your birth partners and midwife.

A birth plan is flexible, and can be altered at any time if you change your mind or your circumstances change. You may decide to add or remove something as you find out more about birth and early parenthood. However it should reflect ideally how you would like to give birth. It may help to write the birth plan with someone – usually your support person in labour. Talking to someone will help give you a clear idea of what you would like and what you would prefer not to have.

You can discuss your birth plan with any of your midwife and/or doctor at any stage in your pregnancy or labour, as they may be able to help you with some of your choices.

Birth Plan of ....

My birth companions will be ....

....

Would you like a student midwife/medical student to support you in labour? Yes ☐ No ☐

Labour equipment

In the room we would like:

A floor mat ☐

Birth ball ☐

Beanbag ☐

Birth Stool ☐

Rebozo ☐

Multitrack ropes ☐

Birth pool ☐

The birth environment

Low lighting ☐

Music ☐

Quiet ☐

Aromatherapy smells ☐

Bed to the side of the room ☐

Quiet voices!!!!! ☐

Positions for labour/birth

- Walk ☐
- Stand ☐
- Kneel ☐
- Squat ☐
- Birth ball ☐
- Birth stool ☐
- Bed ☐

Labour and birth techniques

I am planning on using:

- Hypnobirth techniques ☐
- Surge breathing ☐
- J-breathing ☐
- Birth pool ☐
- I have learnt relaxation techniques ☐
- Massage ☐
- Aromatherapy ☐
- TENS ☐
- Gas and air ☐
- Pethidine/meptid ☐
- Epidural ☐
- ☐
- ☐

After the Birth

I would like the baby to be placed next to my skin immediately after birth ☐

We know the sex of our baby ☐

We would like to discover the sex of our baby ourselves ☐

Who cuts the baby's cord? Mother ☐

Father / Birth Partner ☐

Midwife ☐

I would like to birth the placenta

Naturally without drugs ☐

With assistance using a drug ☐

Our thoughts on vitamin K are ....

....

Any special personal, spiritual or religious needs you may have

....

....

Care plan introduced:	Date	Name	Grade
Early pregnancy			
Care plan discussed:			
36 weeks			
In labour			

Additional information:

Hand Anaesthesia Anchor

Make yourself comfortable and when you are ready you can allow your eyes to gently close.

As your breathing begins to slow down you can allow any tension to drain away as you drift gently down into relaxation. Notice or imagine your feet on the floor, feel how they connect you to the earth and as you breath in you can feel the strong, calm energy of the earth flowing through you, bringing a feeling of strength and confidence.

Take a moment or two now to breathe in deeply and exhale slowly and allow your mind and body to relax. You may be aware of sounds around you, just allow all of these sounds to take you gently, further and further into relaxation.

In a moment I am going to gently stroke the back of your hand and as I continue to stroke your hand and talk to you, you can allow a feeling of numbness, of anaesthesia to develop in your hand. ***[Start stroking the back of her hand]***

As I begin to stroke the back of your hand you can feel yourself relaxing even more, feeling safe and secure, really calm and relaxed. Allowing all sensation to leave your hand now.... of course you know that I'm still stroking your hand, but this feeling of numbness, of anaesthesia gets deeper and deeper. As this feeling deepens and you relax more and more you may be aware sensation, perhaps even tingling as endorphins flow through your body bringing with them a wonderful sense of peace and well-being.

Every time I stroke your hand you drift gently further and further into relaxation, feeling safe and secure and really relaxed. Contd...

Now, as I begin to stroke your arm you can allow that feeling of numbness in your hand to gradually begin to flow up your arm, allowing you to feel more and more relaxed. Allowing that feeling of numbness to travel as far up your arm as you like, so that it's just right for you.

And if you choose, you can move that feeling of numbness to any part of your body, just by thinking about that part of your body and imaging that numbness and anaesthesia flowing there.

Take as much time as you want, resting in this space where time means nothing – an hour seems like a minute. A minute is just a blink. Rest in this space, relax, relax, relax....

[Continue to stroke and when enough time has passed, stop and bring her gently back into the room.]

In a moment it will be time to come back into the room, feeling confident and relaxed, knowing that each time you do this you will find it easier and easier to relax and you will feel more and more confident about the birth of our/your baby. So you can begin by moving your fingers and toes and very gently, in your own time you can gently open your eyes, feeling great.

Home Practice – Week Four

Classes are over! Practice your techniques from now until birth day.

Use your Birth Ball – replace some sofa sitting in the evening with some time spent on the ball. This will put your baby into a great position for birth, alleviate back pain and stretch your inner thighs. All great for birth. If you have not yet bought one – Asda, Tesco and Argos sell them cheaply.

Remind yourselves of **Counting and Breathing,** and **3-Step Touch Breathing.**

Practice Relaxation Breathing – Practice! Practice! Practice! This should be almost second nature by now.

Staircase Deepener – this can be useful at night before sleep. Try it on each other. See how quickly you are teaching your body to relax.

Practice J-Breathing - let's not beat around the bush- the best place to practice is on the toilet. Visualise the downward breath making a J shape as you exhale. Imagine the circular muscles working in perfect coordination to nudge the large object (your baby!) down.

Breath Visualisations – which one does she enjoy most? Finish the day with yoga breath, eye of the storm or ice cube.

Practice Deepening Techniques – shoulder anchor/ hand anaesthesia.

Start thinking about things to include in your birth plan – then write it!

Section EIGHT

Birth Stories

Mandy's story

I came across the concept of Hypnobirthing whilst 3 months pregnant by chance as a friend's granddaughter had recently been born using the method. I had already started thinking about giving birth and I was, in all honesty, very scared by the stories of close friends and family who had all had traumatic experiences.

As soon as we started our first session I knew we had made a good decision. My overactive mind was put at rest from the start as the theory was explained to us. We thoroughly enjoyed each session that followed and I grew in confidence. However it was not until the day our beautiful boy was born that we realised the impact hypnobirthing would have on the birth.

We had prepared for a relaxing few hours of labour, packing snacks, soothing music, books and things to do but when we arrived at the hospital I was almost fully open, having only felt my waters break a couple of hours earlier.

The midwives swiftly moved me to the delivery suite, where I began to feel the overwhelming urge to push.

I wanted a water birth and the midwives had started filling the pool, only to realise that it might not be full in time for the baby to come out. In between my surges I kept asking if it was ready yet and finally they said it was.

It felt wonderful to get into the pool and I distinctly remember a huge grin on my face as I felt the lovely warm water around me. A few minutes later the baby's head was out, and I couldn't believe it as I realised how close I was to

Contd...

holding my baby. One more push and I brought him to the surface with my very own hands. I was so shocked that it was all over and that I hadn't needed pain relief (to be honest, I had forgotten that it was even available!)

My body just seemed to do all the work by itself and I didn't feel any resistance to what was happening. This I can only put down to the trust I had in the capability in my body to do the job it was designed for and my hypnobirth sessions had given me this trust.

Nature is so intelligent and I will never underestimate it again. I gave birth to our baby boy in 2 hours and 45 minutes from the first sign of labour until the time he was born. I never expected that.

Even if we had encountered complications or a long, drawn-out labour, I know our hypnobirth sessions would have gotten us through with a sense that we were in control and that it could still be a calm, relaxing and empowering time.

I recommend hypnobirth to anyone. In fact it seems strange that it should be considered as an 'alternative' way of birthing, as its teachings are only a reminder to our over complicated lives of how birth was always supposed to be, and how it has been for thousands of years before fear came into it and we stopped trusting in our bodies. Thanks to hypnobirth, that magical night when our son was born was the best of our lives.

Alex's story

Having already used similar techniques successfully on a fear of flying course, I knew that relaxation could be used to effectively alleviate fear and at the very least, thought that hypnobirthing might help reduce anxiety in the run up to the birth. I was realistic about its potential to manage pain but any relief would be a bonus! I knew a number of people who had tried hypnobirthing or similar techniques during their labour, albeit using books and/or CDs. All of them said it was worthwhile.

Before I embarked on the course, I had no fixed idea about the type of birth I wanted. I had little understanding of how labour might be impacted by being at home versus being in hospital, what induction involved and how active birth/the use of a pool could help with the speed of delivery and pain. However, I was open minded about the different options available to me. The course (as opposed to the books and CD alone) empowered me to make my own decisions about my birth plan and labour, and gave me confidence that they would be respected by the midwives.

Being a complete first-timer, I found the antenatal content just as useful as the practical exercises. I took a lot from understanding the biological process of pregnancy and birth and used it to inform my birth plan. By the end of the course, I was positively evangelical about natural birth and hypnobirthing.

Although I understood that not all deliveries go to plan, I wanted to avoid intervention as far as possible and opted to have my baby in the midwife led unit (MLU) which I hoped would provide a more relaxing environment and offered

Contd...

the only opportunity (at that time) to use the pool. I just had to keep my fingers crossed that no-one else would be using it at the time!

I was perhaps in a slightly unusual position that my husband did not wish to attend the birth. He is not comfortable in hospitals and we both agreed that it would be better to have someone there who could support me.

Instead, my cousin Syrie acted as my birth partner. She was very experienced after three children of her own but was arguably sceptical about hypnobirthing having never done it herself. Unfortunately, we couldn't rehearse the exercises together between sessions so I listened to the CDs and practiced the breathing every day on my own, mainly when I went to bed.

In the meantime, she planned what she would bring/do to support me based on what I liked best during the sessions, for example, certain types of touch, visualisation and anchoring. I found there were definitely some which I responded to better than others and which I would listen to repeatedly, usually falling asleep before I got to the end!

Despite some initial worries that I wouldn’t be able to find the time to practice every day, I found that it slotted quite easily into my routine.

In fact, I used the techniques on numerous occasions when there was stress at work, on the train home after a hectic day, going to bed and during a procedure to remove an abscess. It was during the latter that I noticed the breathing really helped me manage what was some of the worst pain I have experienced. By the time I was 40 weeks, I was having regular

Contd...

Braxton Hicks and started to use the breathing to get through them.

In order to make my birth space as relaxed as possible, I was encouraged to bring things which would make me comfortable. Examples included a playlist, food and drink and objects to support me during birth. I therefore readied myself with over 76 hours of music, 3 multipacks of Ribena and 3 boxes of Tracker bars; I was clearly expecting a long haul! Syrie also suggested more practical items which she found useful during her own labours and supported an active birth such as a giant bean bag and hot water bottles.

The surges started at 4.30am on the Sunday morning, two curries, many walks and 9 days after my due date. They were markedly more intense than the Braxton Hicks I had experienced over the previous couple of weeks so I had no doubt I was in labour. I started using the breathing and visualisation techniques almost immediately to get through each surge and enjoyed a short bath.

We stayed about 8 hours at home before I decided to go to the hospital with Matthew. At this point Syrie, my birth partner was worryingly incommunicado! In some respects, I wasn't nervous about her being absent if things progressed quickly as I had been practising the breathing on my own so did not feel completely reliant on her. I hadn't felt (and indeed never felt) any fear or anxiety, even as the surges intensified.

The hospital do not do tours so the first time I saw the MLU was in fact when I was in labour. The room with the pool was, thankfully, free so we were shown through and made ourselves at home. I accepted a VE as I was keen to know far

Contd...

along I was. I knew that they could potentially be uncomfortable and slow things down but as I made the decision, I remained relaxed and don't believe it had any impact on progress.

At only 3-4cm I was offered two choices at that stage; to sit it out in the hospital or to head home and come back when the contractions were more frequent/powerful. Although the room was comfortable, it was a little hot and windowless, and still felt quite medicalised so I opted to head home after a dose of liquid painkiller. At the time, I didn't actively think about the impact of this decision but with hindsight it was a good call.

Syrie came over armed with her giant beanbag and hot water bottles and we settled into a small quiet corner of the living room. Completely sub-consciously, I found myself migrating to a more intimate space as had been described during my hypnobirth classes. I largely stayed there for about 5 hours, after which time the surges intensified and I decided it was time to head back to hospital, apparently saying that if they sent me home this time, I wouldn't leave. Syrie said at that point, she knew I was ready!

All the time, I was maintaining my breathing. I could hear Syrie talking to me and I was aware of what was going on around me, but was completely in the moment. I felt happily detached in my own space yet could still talk lucidly to the midwives on the phone and walk comfortably to and from the car. Arguably, I was a bit too lucid. It was only when I explained I was hypnobirthing that the midwives encouraged me to head in!

We got to the hospital at around 7pm. The pool was still free

Contd...

thankfully but I laboured initially in a different room with the beanbag, my music and the hot water bottles! I moved around and breathed through the surges. The shift change roughly coincided with my arrival so I was introduced to my midwife, Cheryl, and her student, Melissa. As it turned out, they would be with me throughout my labour.

Cheryl explained that she was actually a 'high risk' midwife and rarely worked in the MLU so didn't come across hypnobirthing that often. With regular checks from Melissa, she was happy to leave me to it as per my birth plan unless I told her otherwise. A connection is important and I felt immediately comfortable with both of them, especially as they seemed to respect and support my plan. The surges were certainly not pain free by this stage but I focussed on getting through them with breathing and gas and air, knowing that they would pass and with each one I was a step closer to the end.

When a surge was too much and I started to wobble, Syrie brought me back by placing her hands on my shoulders and telling me to relax, using the anchors we had practiced in the sessions. Following a check from Cheryl, we moved across to the pool after about 4 hours. This was a complete revelation! The warm water combined with the breathing provided brilliant pain relief and I was eventually at a point where the gas and air was doing so little, it was simply getting in the way and was mainly ditched.

You always said that we would know when to push and to go with our instinct rather than instruction. I will never forget the change in sensation and reaching down to feel the top of the baby's head before shouting out that I needed to push.

Contd....

There was no warning and it seemed to catch everyone by surprise, myself included.

By this time, I was in an established rhythm of breathing and surges and was unaware (or just ignoring?) conversations going on around me. However, I do remember hearing Cheryl whisper to Syrie that I was only 8cm and had a little way to go. I heard them placing bets on the time she'd be born. I heard Cheryl singing to my playlist. I heard her talk of this mysterious purple line on my back which was apparently significant, although I had never heard of it and had no idea what they were talking about!

My memory of that time was excitement, both myself and in the room, and anticipation that it was all going to happen soon. Perhaps 'soon' was optimistic but I think Cheryl was surprised at how quickly I went from 8cm to fully dilated. There was a lot of back and forth on the baby's part but eventually her head popped out swiftly followed by her shoulders and body. I think talk of her getting stuck and looking at other options (although I don't recall the way it was actually phrased) incentivised her to come out and she obliged on the very next surge!

Constance was born in the water at 4.40am, at least an hour before the midwives and Syrie had predicted and almost exactly 24 hours after the first surges. The feeling is hard to describe but I remember feeling a mixture of euphoria, relief and some anxiety about what lay ahead. Matthew arrived shortly after Connie was born and gave Syrie a well earned rest.

I moved back to the other room and was invited to stay as long as I needed. In the end, we rested in the room until

Contd....

around lunchtime at which point I felt well enough to head home. It was very relaxed and there was no pressure to leave, or indeed move to the postnatal ward upstairs.

I feel blessed to have had a straightforward, natural birth, especially after the experiences of many of my other NCT friends who all had some form of intervention. I admit, some of this was luck; the pool was free, the hospital was quiet, the midwives on shift were great and Syrie was brilliant... However, I truly believe the level of relaxation I was able to achieve during pregnancy and birth was also a significant factor in my positive experience. At no point do I remember feeling fearful or tense, or overwhelmed by pain.

Looking back some months on, I am also increasingly of the belief that a relaxed mum means a relaxed baby. Birth must be one hell of an ordeal at the best of times! However, Connie is one of the happiest, most contented babies I have met. She has eaten and slept well from day one and seems to take everything (including the early emergence of teeth at 4 months!) in her stride. From what I have read subsequently, I am positive that hypnobirthing has contributed in some way to this.

And it doesn't stop at birth. Hypnobirthing is genuinely a skill for life - I have already put it to good use at the dentists!!

Becky's story

My SECOND amazing Hypnobirthing story...

I was given a stretch and sweep on Monday 2nd February (4 days after my "due date"). During the rest of that day I had some mild period type pains. I woke late that night/early hours of Tuesday 3rd February and was having what I would describe as mild surges which were coming regularly every 9-10 minutes and lasting about 1 minute. This went on until about 8am but they then stopped completely. I wasn't concerned and got on with my day (taking a bit of advice from you about how to bring them back on - My special bath bomb and a bit of clary sage oil!!)

I went to bed that night about 11pm and was aware that the surges had started again, but they were completely manageable and in fact I went to sleep. I think I was subconsciously aware of the surges but kept sleeping through them.

By 2.30am I must have subconsciously realised that the surges were getting stronger and closer together because I got up and decided to time them. They were every 5-6 minutes and lasting for about 1 minute. Again the surges were completely manageable and I felt totally in control. I decided that I was so comfortable that the surges would probably stop again so instead of waking Mark I would monitor myself and sit in bed reading - I did this for just under an hour until the surges were getting stronger (although I was still very comfortable and able to talk through them). They were now coming every 4-5 minutes.

I woke Mark about 3.30am and we decided we should call my

Contd...

mum to come and babysit Dexter. I remember joking with her it was probably another false alarm and I was getting her out of bed in her onesie for nothing, but thought we should be on the safe side.

No sooner had I put the phone down that the surges picked up again and were coming every 2 mins, then 4 mins, then 2 mins etc.

I was still really calm and relaxed and told Mark that I wanted to have a shower and wash my hair. Mark was not quite so calm (bless him) and told me this was not an option (thank goodness he took control at that point, he could clearly see how quickly things were progressing!) He was texting someone on his phone and when I asked him who it was he said he was telling my mum to put her foot down because it definitely wasn't a false alarm this time.

My mum arrived about 4am. The surges were every 2-3 minutes by this time and although getting stronger I was still able to breathe through them. I had started using my breathing techniques and visualisations and found it most comfortable to lean on something and rock my pelvis from side to side during the surge.

I had 5 surges during the 15 minute car journey to the hospital and arrived at the hospital around 4.30am.

Our midwife Clare led us to a fantastic birthing room with a POOL!!! I got a birthing pool!!!!

By the time Clare got round to examining me (which was difficult because the surges were now so close together) it was about 4.45am. I was 4cm. My waters were still intact. I wasn't at all disheartened as I knew that for me, given my

Contd....

track record and being a Hypnobirther, this meant our baby would soon be making an appearance.

I was still able to use the breathing techniques to get through the surges and didn't feel the need for any pain relief. I felt controlled and excited at what I knew was about to happen.

I got into the birthing pool around 5am - Wow, it was soooo relaxing! It's an instant pain relief and feels as though all the weight of the baby has been taken from you. I found it to be a huge help.

Clare was very supportive of our Hypnobirthing plan and did not try to intervene or interrupt during the times that she could see I was concentrating. We barely knew she was there. The lights were dimmed and it was a very tranquil environment, just as I had imagined it to be.

By about 5.20am I felt that our baby was coming. I could feel her moving down. I remember at one point reaching down and could feel my water sack which still hadn't broken. With the next surge my waters broke. I believe that I only had about 6 "pushing" surges in total and at 5.45am Jemima made her appearance into the world, weighing 8lb 8oz (exactly 1lb bigger than her brother). In total we were at the hospital for about an hour and a quarter.

It wasn't until near the very end that I felt the need for a little gas and air (I think that may have been because it was all so quick), but I certainly didn't need any other pain relief. The breathing techniques, positive thinking and visualisations were what got me through it. It may sound strange but in my mind I knew that I wouldn't need any sort of intervention because I was so confident about what I had to do, I had

Contd....

planned it in my mind and all I had to do was put it into practice.

Jemima is a very calm, happy baby and it is very rare to hear her cry. She sleeps brilliantly too!! Once again I put this down to Hypnobirthing which kept me relaxed during my pregnancy which clearly transferred on to Jemima.

Both Mark and I are so pleased we decided to do the Hypnobirthing course again, it really made a huge difference. We have been blessed with 2 beautiful children and I have amazing memories of both of their births which I will enjoy sharing with them when they get older. I also love sharing my stories with expecting mums, because unlike so many people who want to tell you about how horrendous their labour was, I have only good things to say about mine and that's the way it should be.

I will continue to recommend Hypnobirthing and you never know if you might see us again on another course!!

Thank you so much for everything you've done for us, you truly are amazing at what you do and are clearly so passionate about hypnobirth. We are so thrilled that we got to meet you and learn from all your knowledge.

Julie's story

I was particularly anxious about the birth this time as my first son Oliver was born by caesarean section. Having seen women cope amazingly through labour in my job as a midwife, I had underestimated the intensity of contractions. Oliver was planned to be born at home but I didn't cope well and coupled with the fact that I didn't dilate terribly quickly I went into hospital for an epidural. Unfortunately my epidural failed to work and, after some bad decision making on my part, I had a caesarean at 3cm dilated.

I was determined that I was not going to have a repeat performance this time and I decided that preparation was the key. I so desperately wanted to achieve a natural birth but mainly I just wanted to cope throughout labour. I attended the hypnobirthing classes and I listened to the CD every night in bed and occasionally in the day – 2 year-old permitting! My husband Kev and I practiced the scripts at weekends when he was home, particularly the shoulder anchoring technique. Because of my previous caesarean I was advised to give birth in hospital. I was very keen for a waterbirth but because I was classed as high-risk this was not an option for me so we negotiated that I would use my own pool at home and we would go to hospital when I felt ready.

I was woken by surges on the Monday morning, 5 days before my due date. They were only coming every 15 minutes so I tried to ignore them as much as possible. I took Ollie to pre-school and spent the morning tidying, doing odd jobs and getting the birthing pool inflated. I picked Ollie up at midday, had lunch and went for a walk. By 3:30pm they were coming every 7 minutes so I called Kev home from work (in

Contd....

Hampshire) and let my Mum know as she was going to care for Ollie for us.

Kev arrived home just before 6pm, we had dinner and put Ollie to bed. At this point my surges were varying between 3-6 minutes. I put my TENS machine on and distracted myself on the birthing ball for a while (I have a new found respect for the Big Bang Theory for keeping me entertained). By 10pm the surges were every 3-4 minutes so I got in the pool (total bliss!) We put some lavender oil in a cup of hot water and played a relaxation CD in the background. I had been experiencing Braxton-Hicks for weeks in the pregnancy and had practiced surge-breathing with them whenever I could. I would picture a white sandy beach with clear blue sea; when I inhaled I would visualise the sun rising and when I exhaled the sun setting. It worked wonderfully with the surges and gave me a real focus.

Kev called the Maternity Unit and Emma came to see me after her late-shift. I felt totally relaxed but if Emma or Kev noticed me tense-up with a surge they applied the shoulder anchor technique which was really effective (to the point that they thought they were going to drown me!). By about 12:15am Emma felt it would be prudent to examine me; I was 2cm dilated. It was at this point in my labour with Ollie that I panicked and went in for an epidural but I took it all in my stride this time. Emma suggested I take paracetamol and go to bed so I put my TENS back on and tucked myself up in bed on my left side.

By 3am the surges were 3 in 10 and much stronger so I got up and mobilised. I didn't want to call Emma or Fiona (midwives on call for me) too early. I contemplated getting back into the

Contd....

pool again but I was starting to think I'd need pain relief soon so I decided to wake Kev and make our way to hospital. Kev started repacking our bags while I made my way downstairs. The surges were 4 in 10 now and by the time Kev was packing the bags in the car I had the distinct urge to push!

Kev rang Emma who kindly rang the hospital and Fiona to let them know I was on my way in. Kev managed to get me on the backseat of the car in between very frequent surges with pushing and I recall a very speedy journey to hospital (I somehow managed to get my seatbelt on whilst lying on my left side with my head in the baby's car-seat). The midwives on Delivery Suite had done a grand job at preparing my birth room. Emma had explained to them that I wanted a cosy homely environment to give birth in so they had removed any non-essential medical equipment from the room, the bed was pushed to the corner in the 'chair-position', there was a beanbag and mat to use, the lights were dimmed and the starry laser-light show was on. Despite all the comfy furnishings I still went and got on the bed!

Fiona arrived 10 minutes after us and she kept the atmosphere calm and relaxed. I could feel he was definitely on his way with the pushes and I wasn't hurried to be examined. My waters broke with one of the surges and a few minutes later I put my hand down and I could feel the top of his head; such relief that he was nearly here! Fiona encouraged me onto my knees leaning over the back of the bed and Kev was really supportive in the loan of his hands to squeeze whilst pushing (they needed a few days to recover). I hadn't practiced the 'J-breathing' much during the pregnancy but it did help at the start of a surge as it built up. However there really is no other way to describe it; you just cannot

Contd....

help but 'push' when the urge is there, your body just does it for you.

At 05:18am Finley was born weighing 7lb 9oz. My established labour was estimated at being only 3 and a half hours long with no drugs at all. Fiona passed him up to me through my legs and we had our first skin to skin cuddle, it was an amazing moment. I had planned to have the syntometrine injection for the 3rd stage after the cord had pulsated for 3 minutes but there were already signs of it separating. I delivered the placenta 8 minutes after Finn was born with very little effort.

Although I couldn't have the waterbirth I wanted, the labour and birth was everything I wished for and more. Never in a million years did I expect to have a quick labour with no drugs culminating in a wonderful natural delivery. I can honestly say I don't think I would have achieved it without employing the techniques of Hypnobirthing. One month on and we have a very chilled out baby and two very proud and happy parents.

Graham's story

Where do we begin with the thank you?

We strongly believe that our experience would not have been possible had it not been for the support and guidance offered by you. The Hypnobirthing classes helped us both to understand the science behind the reality.

Our experience started on Friday afternoon, Kelly was booked in for her fourth and final sweep, prior to being induced. We desperately wanted to have a natural birth and the final sweep was our last chance. The thought of the induction did not scare us but we both felt that this would have robbed us of our experience. So the midwife came around 1:15pm, her words to Kelly were, 'let's get this baby out' certainly words that Kelly wanted to hear.

The midwife hadn't even got off our drive when Kelly started to experience surges, then putting into action all that we had been taught. I was advised to return home from work around 2:30pm. By the time I arrived home, Kelly was walking around the house breathing through the surges, I asked if she wanted to make her way to hospital but this was declined. The surges continued and so did Kelly's breathing, all throughout she had total control of the experience.

After speaking with the hospital at around 3:30 we decided that we should make our way to the hospital, as the surges were grouping nicely. The journey to the hospital was relaxed and calm, I won't lie, this was a surprise to me. Upon arrival at the MLU we were invited to our room, we made ourselves comfortable as the midwife chatted with Kelly regarding our surges. Upon examination we were 5cm, Kelly still breathing

Contd....

through the surges, totally in control, using minimal gas and air.

The surges started to become continuous, one after the other, after the other, we chatted with the midwife and thought that now may be the time to enter the pool. Kelly got into the pool, all the time breathing through the surges, with the occasional pep talk from me regarding controlling the breathing and occasional use of the gas and air.

For 4hrs Kelly experienced surges, breathing, moving and working with the surges. At approximately 8pm Kelly was asked if she wanted a final examination, this was agreed and Kelly was advised that she had escalated to 10cms. Bang on, just through controlling the breathing and shaking the apples in the pool. Kelly advised the midwife of our birthing plan and this was duly accepted. At approximately 8:30pm Kelly got back into the pool, the surges continuing. The midwife keeping a close eye on developments, all the while encouraging Kelly to breathe, along with me offering support to take control of the breathing and own it.

At around 9pm Kelly had birthed the head, we were invited to view. What an amazing experience, the mother in law saw baby looking around and wriggling, Kelly too confirmed the wriggling. The moment that we had both been so excited about was about to become a reality, we were going to have a baby.

The midwife asked me if I was ready to receive the baby, I was, nothing could have stopped me from receiving our baby and handing it to Kelly. I was a little nervous, but after looking into Kelly's eyes I knew everything was going to be ok, Kelly moved and I took the baby from her and slowly, lifted it from

Contd....

the water to find out we had had a baby girl. I handed her to Kelly, who, after all of her comments during the classes regarding the cleaning of the baby after birth, immediately kissed her. We were and are the proud parents of a healthy baby girl, Isla-Mai and I couldn't be more proud of my wife, to show the strength and control through the birth and I strongly believe that had we not done the hypnobirth classes this would have been a different story.

The whole experience was as rewarding as we wanted it to be and I would like to thank you from the bottom of my heart for assisting us throughout our pregnancy.

Go hypnobirth!

Rachel's story

I knew from the beginning that I wanted to fully immerse myself in the experience of being pregnant, and the birthing of our baby. In the early stages of pregnancy I was frequently amazed and in awe of what our bodies are capable of, and the wonder of growing a baby. I had a clear idea of how I hoped to birth our child, and this spurred me to research the possibility of practicing the methods relating to hypnobirth. After reading several articles and watching YouTube videos about the benefits and positive outcomes of hypnobirth, Chris and I found a course. The course was everything we hoped and provided us with the knowledge, techniques and confidence to approach birth in a positive and relaxed manner.

Sunday 15th February early morning I awoke to mild back pain but thought very little of it, at 9.15am my waters broke after a lazy snooze on the sofa! After being examined at triage by Charlotte a very lovely midwife, to confirm my waters had actually broken, followed by a sweep - in which Charlotte felt our baby's mass of hair, we ventured to Waitrose to buy food for our hospital bag. At this stage there were still no surges but my waters continued to leak. I was becoming increasingly concerned that my surges wouldn't start and induction would be planned for the following morning. I rang our midwife Teri and she advised me to use my breast pump for nipple stimulation to gently encourage my labour to progress, also to continue to be mobile and active.

On returning home I started to feel mild cramping sensation in my lower stomach which I was most pleased about!! I had

Contd....

a bath and began to focus on relaxation and preparing my body for what was to follow. Our class relaxation CD and clary sage essential oil in my diffuser really helped me to focus and relax. As my surges began to intensify slowly I used my birthing ball for comfort, rocking back and forth really helped with the increasing sensation in my back and lower stomach.

I also found at this time that a hot water bottle placed on my lower back, and starting to focus on my breathing with Chris really helped a great deal. I felt so ready and relaxed, as the surges became more frequent I was able to focus and breathe my way through them with ease.

Around 5 pm Chris made dinner and encouraged me to eat and drink. At this time my surges were becoming more frequent and I found comfort in leaning on the kitchen work surface whilst Chris timed the duration of the surges, ate his dinner, massaged my back and helped me focus on my breathing! After a phone call to Teri updating her on timings and progress she advised us to continue to stay at home until I was reaching 4 surges in 10 minutes. Staying active and mobile really helped with my progress, and being in the comfort of my own home, in familiar surroundings was deeply reassuring.

At 8pm we made our way to the hospital, Chris rang ahead to let them know we were on our way. My sister drove us and has subsequently said how quiet and focused we both were with no sense of drama or anxiety. She was surprised by the intense focus and connection to what was happening, and my ability to maintain control. I felt completely calm, with my surges continuing throughout the 15 minute journey, of which I remember very little. . I was unaware that my surges

Contd....

were still present and expressed a concern to Chris that they had stopped, he assured me that they hadn't as he had witnessed my body still responding, but I couldn't recall the sensation as my mind was focused elsewhere.

At 8.15pm we arrived at the hospital and Teri had also made her way in too, the welcoming birthing room and Teri's presence made me feel instantly safe, calm and ready for birth. I believe my oxytocin levels at this point were high due to this perfect environment which enabled me to cancel out fear and anxiety. After examination I discovered I was 9cm dilated. As I continued to breathe through the surges with some sacral massage from Teri, the birthing pool was filled, the lights dimmed and the star projector created an amazing calming effect that filled the room. I felt safe and ready. Chris placed our LED candles around the space and the relaxation music used in class was played on my iPod.

The pool was both comforting and strangely euphoric; the warm water had such a soothing affect on my body I instantly let go of any tension. My surges were increasing steadily and I was approaching the next stage of labour. Both Teri and Chris were supportive and tentative, but in a quiet and peaceful manner remaining present, but allowing me to concentrate. It was at this point that I instinctively used the anchoring techniques learnt in class, using Chris' hand on my forehead as a point of strength and focus. The feeling of intense pressure, and a change in rhythm with regards to my surges, meant that the final stage was approaching, and my body felt as if it was starting to work harder to birth our baby. This feeling was strangely satisfying, and with the use of J breathing and a centred humming sound, I focused all my efforts down.

Contd....

I never once believed that I was incapable of birthing our baby, and the use of any pain relief didn't even enter my head. I felt confident and determined with a deep sense of trust in my body and baby. Reaching forward and feeling my baby's head in the final stage of labour gave me that last rush of determination and strength. At 10.11pm Winnie arrived. Eased out of the water by Chris, with her eyes open and with a sense of serenity and wonder. Winnie was placed on my chest and lifted her head to focus on my face. This moment was intensely emotional and one I will never forget. I couldn't believe she was finally here, and I couldn't believe what I had achieved!!

After learning about the benefits of delaying the clamping of the umbilical cord, we decided to wait and allowed the cord to stop pulsating; following this Chris finally cut the cord.

We are so proud at what we achieved with regards to Winnie's birth, and we are proud to have been part of a hypnobirth learning experience. We continuously share our positive birth story, and feel passionate about encouraging others to change their thoughts surrounding child birth. I cannot recommend the hypnobirth course enough, and urge any expectant parents to go along and feel enlightened, confident and empowered.

I look back on my birth as a truly positive, empowering and amazing experience; I believe that Winnie's contented nature, my swift labour and peaceful birth is a product of our commitment to the hypnobirthing preparation and techniques – teamed with support from an inspirational midwife and teacher, outstanding birthing facilities, and exceptional antenatal care.

Vicky's story

Firstly I wanted to thank you for the fantastic experience of the hypnobirthing class. I remember how hearing you reading other people's experiences out in class really helped me so I thought I'd send you mine. I think it will help people to know how hypnobirthing can help even when things get a little intense!

Gareth and I welcomed our little Molly into the world on Easter Monday at 4:15am.

During the week before I'd been getting random period type cramps sporadically and kept thinking "is this it?" But nothing came of them. Most of the time I just needed to use the toilet and then the cramps went away!

On Easter Sunday we had dinner with my family, as I got up to drive home at 8pm I had another cramp. The best way to describe it is a cross between a period pain and an upset stomach. We drove home and got back half an hour later, I'd had no more cramps so I thought it was the same as the rest.

When I got in I had another pain so decided to go and have a bath. I had no more pain in the bath so stayed there for about 40 minutes. When I got out of the bath at 10pm I felt another intense cramp and realised that they were in fact surges and that things were starting.

Straight away my surges came fast and intense, they were very irregular but close together, starting at 5 minutes apart, going to 2 minutes then 3, then 1 then back to 5 and they varied in length and intensity.

We called the hospital because they were close together but

Contd....

irregular and were told to wait until they were 3 every 10 minutes and so regular in distance and length that you could set your watch by them.

I admit after about 2 hours I had a little wobble, I found the surges very intense and was vomiting with some of them so couldn't keep down any Paracetemol. I thought that after a couple of hours I was probably only 1-2cm dilated and I thought I couldn't cope with it for another 10+ hours.

Gareth calmed me down with the soft touch massage and we put on the relaxation CD so I could use that to focus my breathing. It really helped to get me back on track.

We phoned the hospital again and were again told that they weren't regular but we could come in if we wanted to.

Suddenly at about 2:15am I had an urge to push. We grabbed our stuff and went to the car, then things got very intense very quickly. I was pushing so much that Gareth thought we may give birth in the car!

At the hospital we couldn't get into the ward, I think because we hadn't called ahead. It took a while for someone to let us in, I wanted to be on all fours so I was doing that in the hospital corridor waiting for someone to let us in!

Once I was in the delivery suite I had another surge and my waters released, my midwife ran the birth pool and examined me and I was 10cm dilated!!

Needless to say I didn't make it into the pool! By the time it had run I was too in the zone to move. I stayed on all fours on a bean bag and focused on my breathing, Gareth maintained the soft touch massage. 55 minutes after arriving at hospital

Contd....

Molly was born, she came out so fast that my midwife didn't catch her, she said Molly was "like a cork out of a bottle!"

My placenta was managed, I tried to do it myself but it wouldn't come, so the midwife helped.

I suffered a 3rd degree tear and needed surgery to repair but had to wait another 6 hours for the surgeon to see me so again I used my breathing to help keep me calm whilst we waited.

I know it all sounds quite dramatic but my point to all this is that I managed to birth Molly completely naturally with absolutely no pain relief. Looking back I now believe there is no way I could have done this without hypnobirth. I was able to stay home right until the end and even breathe myself through my tear. When I felt hypnobirth wasn't working it was because I thought I was barely dilated, but in fact I'd breathed my way through the whole birth!

Speaking to Gareth, he found the whole experience completely empowering, he was able to support me the whole way through and it felt like a very intimate experience (our midwife gave us lots of space and with me being on all fours I barely saw her!) it felt like it was just me and Gareth and I had complete trust in him to help me through my surges. He in turn felt very involved with the birth.

My experience is that even when it all felt too intense I was able to stop and collect myself using the techniques you taught us.

I'm so thankful that I did the hypnobirth class. An hour after my surgery I was talking to Gareth about the next baby!

Straight away I knew I could do that again!

Lucy's story

Having had a slightly complicated induction with our first daughter Chloe in 2012 we decided to enrol on the hypnobirth classes for baby number two, due June 2015.

The classes were brilliant and they put all our fears and worries to rest. We did plenty of relaxation practice at home and decided on a home birth too. At 4am on Monday 8th June my waters broke. My surges began immediately but were irregular and gentle so I decided to stay in bed and tried to get back to sleep! An hour or two passed and I decided to wake my husband as I was getting excited!

At 7am my Mum collected my daughter as my surges were becoming slightly more intense. At 8am I rang the midwife to just make them aware that I had started my labour. I put some lavender in a bowl of hot water to relax me and at 10am a midwife and student midwife visited us, by which time I was bouncing on my birth ball and using the breathing techniques I had learnt to get through the surges which were still pretty irregular.

The midwife asked if I'd like to be examined but I said I knew I wasn't particularly far along so didn't want to be 'put off' by an internal examination and she was supportive of my decision. They left and I said I would ring later once things progressed.

At 11am my husband and I went back to bed and at noon I woke to more intense and regular surges! At this point I had a feeling I wasn't far away from delivery so we called the midwife, closed the curtains put our relaxation CD on and put the lights down low. My husband filled the birth pool whilst

Contd....

I sniffed a tissue that had a few drops of clary sage on it and by this time I was instinctively calm but vocal – making a slight humming sound during surges which took me and my husband by surprise, but it was working a treat and I took myself off to another place using the visualisations I had learnt.

When I got in the pool it was like a huge weight had been lifted and I relaxed even more. Shortly after 1pm the same midwife and student midwife arrived and not long after that I had an overwhelming urge to breathe my baby out, and again I was pretty vocal and did not open my eyes as I didn't want to break my concentration. A third midwife was called to assist and it was the midwife that I had seen for every antenatal appointment which was fantastic and I was so happy to see her.

I slowly gave birth to my baby girl Amelia at 2.22pm using the 'J' breathing technique and I could not be prouder! She weighed 8lbs 10oz! Now two weeks on I feel recovered and so grateful that we had the birth we had planned!

Marianne's story

I was told that the baby "was a good size" and I was 5 days overdue. I had a few tightenings but nothing major, I put it down to Braxton Hicks.

I went to the doctors for a sweep on the 19th November and the midwife informed me that I was already 3 cm dilated. I didn't think anything of it being my first pregnancy. Later on in the evening, about 9pm, I felt what I would describe as mild period pain and back ache. I still didn't think that it was labour. I called the MLU (Midwifery Led Unit) and they said stay at home. I had a warm bath, a cup of tea, and got into bed. At 1am I'd say that's when the surges started to kick in but were really manageable. I started to time them at this point. I called the hospital again and they still didn't believe I was in established labour.

At 3.40 am I woke Nick up, breathing through very strong surges and said I think we need to go to hospital. We put the bags and car seat in the car and expected to be sent home. I was that relaxed that I drove to the hospital, having 3 or 4 surges every 10 minutes.

When we arrived we were given a delivery room, I was shocked when the midwife said that I was 6cm. This was about 4.30am. By 7am I was fully open. The baby was back to back and very painful, the surges were manageable but I did have gas and air.

At 7am I got into the birth pool and that was amazing, nice and dark room and my new midwife was brilliant and very understanding of hypnobirth. She reminded me to breathe and not push.

Contd....

I could feel the baby's head come down and up, down and up, just as you said, and down and it stayed where it was..... The point of no return!! We didn't use the scripts as everything happened so quickly but the relaxing, zoning out and listening to my body and breathing really worked. Just breathing, the head crowned and was out. Then the shoulders, then the rest of the baby. I put my hands down and caught our daughter. It was amazing

Thanks to the hypnobirth classes, Nick knew everything that was happening and never felt like a spare part. We have a calm baby, who rarely cries

Johanna weighed in at a whopping 9lb 10, 1 1/2 lb bigger than anyone thought. I had NO stitches or tears. The labour was 4 hours 14 mins, wasn't established labour until 3.30am. I am quite slim and never thought a baby of that size would ever fit through me, let alone doing it naturally. It was the most empowering experience of my life. I can't wait to do it again... I've got to work my magic on Nick though hahaha!

Lisa's Story

It was about 10:30pm and I was watching a comedy in bed. There was a loud pop and my waters went with a gush. It was the night before my due date. This was also how my waters went with my first born, late at night in bed, only this time they weren't nice and clear but green. My heart sank. I was worried and scared. My husband spoke to the birthing centre, my choice for labour, and as I expected they told me I now had go to hospital. Four changes of trousers later (I never would have guessed there would be so much water that just keeps coming) and several phone calls later to get childcare for my son we were on our way to hospital.

The drive to hospital was about 30min or so, to be honest I can't really remember it. My husband put on our hypnobirth CD and as surges started I tried to relax and think positively. The meconium was really worrying me. Arriving at hospital at about midnight we were informed that they were very busy and had no beds in delivery so I was taken to a prenatal ward and monitored. This meant being strapped to a machine having baby's heart rate and my surges monitored. The surges seemed to be getting stronger and closer together. I was very pleased about this as in contrast to my first labour I had to be induced as my surges didn't get going for nearly 48 hours. That said it was at about this time that the midwife informed me I would have to be induced this time too because of the meconium and risk that poses for baby. Having been induced before I knew what this meant but also knew I could cope.

Monitoring continued and I tried my hardest to ignore my worries over the meconium and stayed and I hoped my surges would speed up so that I might avoid the dreaded

Contd....

induction. However, at about 2:30am I went down to the delivery suite and the drip was administered. I can't remember how frequent my surges were at this point but I was coping well with them. One midwife commented that she hoped when she had a baby she would be like me in labour as I seemed so relaxed. This one little comment was a much needed, massive boost to my confidence. I was doing ok!

At this point I was hooked up and having my surges and baby's heart rate monitored and also the induction drip. I was also having gas and air by this point too. It gave me a focus during a surge. I was mostly standing, swaying holding my husband's hands. I also had a birthing ball and chair to sit on but nothing was really helping me get comfortable and I felt very limited being hooked up to a machine. It made moving very difficult and I wanted to walk around. My movement kept moving the monitors on my tummy and after some discussion with the MW I agreed to have a monitor put on the baby's head. I was hesitant in having this as I was worried it might hurt baby or scar her head but was reassured and also told it would mean I would be able to move more. This was not the case as my surges intensified and became closer together, I can't remember what was said, or how it happened but I ended up on the bed lying on my left side and told that the baby was much happier with me in this position. I think it was when they put the monitor on baby's head. It was also at about this time I was given a stomach acid neutralising pill and told 'we are giving them to all our high risk ladies' to me this only meant one thing - they were getting me ready for a c section. I have a massive fear of a c section and mentally told myself this was not happening and that baby was going to come NOW. I think within about

Contd....

30-40min of taking this pill our daughter was born. Things moved very quickly. The surges seemed to be coming more and more frequently and stronger and stronger. I reached a point where I thought I couldn't do it anymore. It was around here that I knew I was close and had to use all my strength to stay calm and relaxed. I had to dig deep however to keep my focus and every ounce of energy I had I used to stay calm and relaxed. I found this very hard to do.

I felt the baby's head very clearly move down and remember thinking how different it felt from my son's birth. My perineum had been numbed in preparation to be cut when I gave birth to my son (thankfully this didn't happen this time) I never actually felt him being born. As I didn't have anything to compare this too I thought that was normal. This time however I could feel everything and it came as a surprise. My husband had to hold my leg up as I had no energy to do this. The head moving down. My skin stretching. A burning sensation as the head began to emerge. A strong urge to just give one really big push to stop the horrid burning sensation that seemed to be going on for a very long time. Something I resisted as I knew it was better for my body to do it slowly. I stayed relaxed and calm and trusted my body that it knew what to do.

Timings of events are very blurred for me as my whole focus was on relaxing and staying calm. My husband tells me this last stage from when I told the MW 'the baby is coming' (which was when I first felt her head move down) and to our daughter being born was about 5 minutes. For me it seemed to take a long time yet be very quick all at the same time. The time was 6am. She was beautiful, calm and perfectly well.

Contd....

I don't remember her crying. My relaxed, controlled way meant I didn't tear. I had the injection for the third stage and then spent the next hour or 2 having wonderful skin to skin. After 12 hours of monitoring we came home as both my daughter and I were well and happy.

Jodi's story

I attended your classes with my husband James and I thought I'd email you the great news that we had our baby. We've named her Sophia. My birth was absolutely wonderful and I know that without your help things would have been much more different. I can't thank you enough for your support, help and everything you did.

Before attending your hypnobirthing class I was determined to have a c-section and as many drugs as available. I can't believe I had a natural birth and I enjoyed every moment.

Here's my hypnobirthing story....

When I fell pregnant my midwife visited and asked what type of birth I wanted. I responded with 'drugs' and a 'c section'. When she asked why, I explained I was terrified of birth and I had a low pain threshold. I felt a mixed bag of emotions. I felt guilty that I was scared of bringing my child in to the world. I felt scared (after all so many people had shared their horror story with me). I also felt powerless as no one knew how the birth would go. My midwife suggested hypnobirth lessons and I agreed.... soon I realised that labour and birth didn't need to be a horrible, daunting and painful experience.

On Tuesday evening I felt some surges. I breathed through them and because they weren't painful I assumed it was Braxton Hicks. I stayed downstairs watching movies timing the surges during the night. At first they were every 17 minutes, then reducing down to 10 minutes, 8 minutes.... And by 4am I realised the surges were every 3 minutes.

I made some toast with raspberry jam on and coffee and I

Contd....

took it up to my husband who was asleep and I told him that 'I think I'm in labour... but it doesn't hurt!?!'

I had a shower, whist he ate his toast, and I stayed very calm breathing through the surges.

On the way to the hospital I called the ward and was told that I should have called before I left home as I probably wouldn't have needed to come in. They said that as I was nearly at the hospital that I should go in but warned I would probably be sent home.

As I walked in to the hospital I reminded myself how the smell of the hospital resembled 'Life' and 'healing'.

When I arrived in the MLU I was asked to take a seat. After ten minutes I went into a birthing suite. I was chatting to the midwife and used the birthing ball to ease my surges. In fact the birthing ball eased them completely. The midwife told me it was highly unlikely that I was in labour as I wouldn't have been able to have a conversation if I was and I would be (as she demonstrated) bent over the bed unable to speak.

I was a bit disappointed and braced myself to go home. The midwife did an examination and to our astonishment she found I was 2cm dilated.

I stayed in the birthing room feeling very relaxed and within 45 minutes I wanted to push. My husband called the midwife who examined me again. I was now 10cm dilated but I was not feeling any pain. I was offered gas and air which I took (mainly because I was a little nervous).

I stayed in stage 2 of my birth for 22 minutes. There was not

Contd....

enough time to fill the birthing pool and instead I gave birth on all fours.

It's incredibly embarrassing to say but a big worry for me was that I pooped during the birth and that is exactly what I thought I had done... I was devastated and said to the midwife how sorry I was. The midwife assured me that I hadn't and instead it was the head which I had delivered.

I couldn't believe it!

It was unbelievable that it was nearly over. All those months of worry and it was a pain free and a wonderful birth. I wish I had enjoyed my pregnancy more and stopped stressing over the birth.

Hypnobirth was incredible and a massive contributing factor in to how I was home within 10 hours of arriving in to the hospital. I cannot thank you enough or explain how much this has been life changing. Thank you.

Section NINE

Reading List, Resources and References

Reading List

Ina May's Guide to Childbirth by **Ina May Gaskin –** Vermilion 2003

Spiritual Midwifery by **Ina May Gaskin –** Book Publishing Company 1975

Childbirth without Fear: **Grantly Dick-Read** – Pinter and Martin 2004

Gentle Birth, Gentle Mothering: A Doctor's Guide to Natural Childbirth and Gentle Early Parenting Choices by **Sarah Buckley** – Celestial Arts, New York. 2009

New Active Birth: A Concise Guide to Natural Childbirth by **Janet Balaskas –** Thorsons 2012

The Birth Partner: A Complete Guide to Childbirth for Dads, Doulas, and Other Labor Companions by **Penny Simkin –** The Harvard Common Press 2008

Birth Pain power to transform- a guide for pregnant women. **Verena Schmid** – Fresh Heart Publishing 2011

The Oxytocin Factor. **Kerstin Uvnas Moberg** – Da Capo Press 2003

Resources

Support and information about maternity choices in the UK

www.aims.org.uk

www.birthrights.org.uk

www.rcog.org.uk/en/patients/patient-leaflets

www.nice.org.uk/guidance

Information/preparation during pregnancy

www.spinningbabies.com

www.dancingforbirth.com

www.activebirthcentre.com/

www.oneworldbirth.net/

www.placentanetwork.com

Induction of labour

www.apps.who.int/rhl/pregnancy_childbirth/induction/en/index.html

www.sarawickham.com/

www.aims.org.uk/

www.nice.org.uk/guidance/cg70

Skin to skin contact/Breastfeeding

www.unicef.org.uk/BabyFriendly/Health-Professionals/Care-Pathways/Breastfeeding/Birth/

www.bestbeginnings.org.uk/fbtb

Rebirth/bonding

www.southwalesdoulas.co.uk/blog/2014/11/08/The-Rebirthing-Ceremony-Validating-our-Grief.aspx

References

Adachi K, Shimada M, Usui A. *The relationship between the parturient's positions and perceptions of labor pain intensity.* Nursing Research. 2003 Jan-Feb;52(1):47-51.

Bourne (2014) www.vagendamagazine.com

Dick-Read G. (2004) *Childbirth without Fear.* London: Pinter and Martin

Davidson, R.J. & Begley, S. (2012). *The Emotional Life of Your Brain.* New York: Hudson Street Press.

Eason, E., Labrecque, M., Wells, G., Feldman, P. Preventing perineal trauma during childbirth: a systematic review. *Obstetrics and Gynaecology.* 2000 Mar: 95 (3): 464-71

Green J,M (1993) *Expectations and experiences of pain in labor: findings from a large prospective study* Birth Jun;20(2):65-72

Krasner, A. (1990/1991). *The Wizard Within.* Irvine, CA: American Board of Hypnotherapy Press.

Labrebcque, M., Eason, E., Marcoux, S. Women's views on the practice of prenatal perineal massage. *British Journal of Obstetrics and Gynaecology.* 2001 May: Vol 108 (5) 499-504.

Lewis, G (ed) (2007). *The Confidential Enquiry into Maternal and Child Health (CEMACH). Saving Mothers' Lives: reviewing maternal deaths to make motherhood safer-* 2003-2005. The Seventh Report on Confidential Enquiries into Maternal Deaths in the United Kingdom. London: CEMACH.

Mead, M (1928) Coming of age in Samoa: A Psychological Study of Primitive Youth for Western Civilisation. Harper Collins New York.

Mikiel-Kostyra K, Mazur J, Bołtruszko,I. (2002). Effect of early skin-to-skin contact after delivery on duration of breastfeeding: a prospective cohort study. *Acta Paediatr* , 91(12):1301-6.

National Institute for Health and Care Excellence (NICE) 2014 *Intrapartum care: care of healthy women and their babies during childbirth*

Odent M. (2007) *Birth and breastfeeding: rediscovering the needs of women during pregnancy and childbirth.* Clairview Books

Odent M. 2002 *The First Hour Following Birth: Don't Wake the Mother!* http://www.midwiferytoday.com/articles/firsthour.asp

Royal College of Obstetricians and Gynaecologists (2014) *Clamping of the umbilical cord and placental transfusion.* Scientific Impact Paper No. 14 February 2015

Schmid, V. (2011) *Birth Pain – Explaining sensations, exploring possibilities.* Fresh Heart Publishing, Chester Le Street

Shipman, M.K., Boniface, D.R., Tefft , M.E. , McCloghry, F. Antenatal perineal massage and subsequent perineal outcomes: a randomised controlled trial. *British Journal of Obstetrics and Gynaecology* 1997 Jul: 104(7): 787-91

Sutton, J. & Scott, P. (1996). *Understanding and Teaching Optimal Foetal Positioning* . Tauranga, New Zealand: Birth Concepts.

Thangamuthu A, Russell IF, Purva M (2013). Epidural failure rate using a standardised definition. *International Journal of Obstetric Anesthesia* 22(4):310-315

Uvnas-Moberg, K (2003) *The Oxytocin Factor: Tapping the Hormone of Calm, Love and Healing*. London: Pinter and Martin

Wickham, S (2014) www.sarawickham.com